WG
300
CON

Adult basic life support

Check responsiveness   Shake and shout

WITHDRAWN

This book is due for return on or before the last date shown below.

5 DEC 2002   17 NOV 2014

0 8 MAY 2003   13/10/16

26 MAY 2004

22 NOV 2004

10 FEB 2005
19 MAY 2005

20 OCT 2005

21 AUG 2006

- 3 NOV 2006

14 DEC 2007
3 - JUN 2008
2 2 MAR 2010

26 APR 2011

D0492452

www.harcourt-international.com

Bringing you products from all Harcourt Health Sciences companies including Baillière Tindall, Churchill Livingstone, Mosby and W.B. Saunders

- ◉ **Browse** for latest information on new books, journals and electronic products

- ◉ **Search** for information on over 20 000 published titles with full product information including tables of contents and sample chapters

- ◉ **Keep up to date** with our extensive publishing programme in your field by registering with eAlert or requesting postal updates

- ◉ **Secure online ordering** with prompt delivery, as well as full contact details to order by phone, fax or post

- ◉ **News** of special features and promotions

If you are based in the following countries, please visit the country-specific site to receive full details of product availability and local ordering information

USA: www.harcourthealth.com

Canada: www.harcourtcanada.com

Australia: www.harcourt.com.au

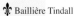 Baillière Tindall CHURCHILL LIVINGSTONE Mosby W.B. SAUNDERS

Evidence-based
MANUAL OF CORONARY CARE MANAGEMENT

Commissioning Editor: Miranda Bromage
Project Development Manager: Paul Fam
Senior Project Manager: Helen Sofio

Evidence-based
MANUAL OF CORONARY CARE MANAGEMENT

Mark Connaughton BA MBBS MRCP MD
Department of Cardiology
South West Cardiothoracic Centre
Derriford Hospital, Plymouth

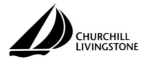

London • Edinburgh • New York • Philadephia • St. Louis • Sydney • Toronto 2001

CHURCHILL LIVINGSTONE
An imprint of Harcourt Publishers Limited

© Harcourt Publishers Limited 2001

 is a registered trademark of Harcourt Publishers Limited

The right of Mark Connaughton to be identified as author of this work has been asserted
by him in accordance with the Copyright, Designs and Patents Act 1988

ISBN 0443 06415 6
Published 2001
  Reprinted 2001

British Library Cataloguing in Publication Data
A catalogue record for this book is available from the British Library

Library of Congress Cataloging in Publication Data
A catalog record for this book is available from the Library of Congress

Note
Medical knowledge is constantly changing. As new information becomes available, changes
in treatment, procedures, equipment and the use of drugs become necessary. The author
and the publisher have, as far as it is possible, taken care to ensure that the information given
in this text is accurate and up to date. However, readers are strongly advised to confirm
that the information, especially with regard to drug usage, complies with latest
legislation and standards of practice.

Existing UK nomenclature is changing to the system of Recommended International
Nonproprietary Names (rINNs). Until the UK names are no longer in use, these more
familiar names are used in this book in preference to rINNs, details of which may be
obtained from the British National Formulary.

The
publisher's
policy is to use
**paper manufactured
from sustainable forests**

Typeset by IMH(Cartrif), Loanhead. Scotland
Printed in China by RDC Group Limited
C/02

To Linda, Charlie and Olivia

For all the time I could have spent with you

Contents

This manual is written primarily for doctors in post-graduate training posts involved in the acute management of patients on hospital coronary care units (CCUs). A background knowledge of acute medicine and competence with practical procedures has been assumed on the basis that the doctor will have at least 1–3 years post-qualification experience in acute internal medicine or in cardiology. It is assumed that while a wide range of non-invasive investigations will be available, facilities such as coronary angiography will not be available in the admitting hospital.

The manual's intention is to give state-of-the-art advice on CCU patient management based on currently available evidence and working practices. To help achieve this it has several novel features: it is formatted so that the left-hand pages can be used as a stand-alone guide to patient management; further explanation, background information and detailed references are given on the right-hand pages. Care has been taken to provide sources not only of the evidence underlying the recommendations given, but also of the quality of that evidence. Management recommendations are in line with the National Service Framework for Coronary Heart Disease in England. Checklists are contained in relevant sections to allow rapid review of whether the relevant tasks have been completed in an individual's management. These are easily adaptable for different hospital settings.

The style is deliberately didactic. The basis for this approach is that in a difficult or emergency situation clear advice is almost always superior to woolly instructions to 'consider' a list of potential options. It is recognised that many experienced clinicians will disagree with certain of the recommendations and the basis for them. It is also accepted that many of the recommendations will require adjustment in the light of local circumstances and facilities. Where this is particularly likely to be the case this has been indicated in the main text.

The manual sets out to be as useable and practical as possible. In the real world, an over busy on-call doctor will find counsels of perfection tiresome and unrealistic. The prime aim is to provide clear guides to patient management for the vast majority of problems CCU doctors will face, with pointers towards the rationale and justification for these treatment plans. If this guide helps to 'bail out' relatively inexperienced doctors when on the CCU, provides them with useable facts and evidence, and helps make their treatments consistently closer to acknowledged standards of excellence, it will more than have achieved its purpose.

I am very grateful to the many experienced cardiologists, nurses and technical experts who have shared their expertise during the writing of this manual, especially those who have commented on drafts of the manuscript. My sincere thanks are due particularly to Professor Douglas Chamberlain, Professor Keith Fox, Professor John Hampton, Dr Andrew McLeod, Dr Andrew Marshall, Dr Howard Marshall, Dr

André Ng, Dr Jim Shahi, Dr David Smith, Dr John Townend, Sr Claire Roberts, Sr Jayne Tarplin and Mr Andrew Lane. I am grateful to Julie Taylor for substantial assistance with the proof reading. Any outstanding errors remain my own.

The author would welcome any criticisms, suggestions or updates, particularly when these could be incorporated in any future editions.

Mark Connaughton
2001

Left hand pages – give management advice – 'what do I do now?' – with little background information.

Right hand pages – give background information – 'why is that done?' including clinical trial evidence, and recommendations from expert consensus guidelines. The following were regarded as key secondary sources, regrettably there are no recent UK guidelines of similar depth.

Quoted in text as	Full references
ACC/AHA	Ryan, TJ et al, (1996) ACC/AHA guidelines for the management of patients with acute myocardial infarction: a report of the American College of Cardiology/American Heart Association Task Force on Practice Guidelines *J Am Coll Cardiol* 28;1328–1428 Ryan, TJ et al[(1999) The 1999 update: ACC/AHA guidelines for the management of patients with acute myocardial infarction *J Am Coll Cardiol* 1999 34:890-911 Full text guidelines available at: www.acc.org www.americanheart.org
Euro	The Task Force on the management of acute myocardial infarction of the European Society of Cardiology (1996) Acute myocardial infarction: pre-hospital and in-hospital management *Eur Heart J* 17:43-63 Full text is available at wwwescardio.org/scinfol guidelines.htm
Thompson	Thompson, PL (Ed.) (1997) Coronary Care Manual Churchill Livingstone: New York ISBN 0 443 052 328

Large clinical trials have been referred to by their acronyms (e.g. ISIS–2, GUSTO) and are referenced separately. Other references are given in full in the text.

Quality of evidence

A welcome recent trend is that the quality of evidence influencing clinical practice is often assessed in reviews. The ACC/AHA rating system is frequently referred to within this manual.

Class I: Conditions for which there is evidence and/or general agreement that a given procedure or treatment is beneficial, useful and effective.

Class II: Conditions for which there is conflicting evidence and/or a divergence of opinion about the usefulness/efficacy of a procedure or treatment.

Class IIa: Weight of evidence/opinion is in favour of usefulness/efficacy

Class IIb: Usefulness/efficacy is less well established by evidence/opinion

Class III: Conditions for which there is evidence and/or general agreement that a procedure/treatment is not useful/effective and in some cases may be harmful.

Recommendations within the manual are drawn only from Class I and Class IIa indications.

The following scheme has been used to rate evidence and treatment recommendations:

i ratings for evidence

(✓✓✓)
Large randomised controlled trials
Systematic reviews
Meta-analysis
Class I AHA/ACC recommendations

(✓✓)
Smaller randomised controlled trials
Large registries
Retrospective analysis from large databases
Limited reviews including editorials
Class IIa AHA/ACC recommendations
European Society of Cardiology recommendations

(✓)
Observational studies
Small series
Other sources of evidence not considered above

ii ratings for treatment recommendations

(✪✪✪)
Based directly on ✓✓✓ evidence
Based directly on established physiology
Likely to be life-saving
Few or no other treatment options exist
note: all recommendations in **bold type** can be assumed to be ✪✪✪

(✪✪)
Extrapolated from ✓✓✓ evidence
Based directly on ✓✓ evidence
Extrapolated from established physiology

(✪)
Extrapolated from ✓✓ evidence
Based directly on ✓ evidence
Traditional or reasonable practice not based on trial evidence

Useful websites

This is a very rapidly expanding field and only a relatively small number of key sites are listed. An extensive list can be found on the European Society of Cardiology website at www.escardio.org.

Journals

Bandolier	www.jr2.ox.ac.uk/bandolier
BMJ	www.bmj.com
Circulation	circ.ahajournals.org
Clinical Cardiology	clinical-cardiology.org
Evidence-based Cardiovascular Medicine	www.churchillmed.com/Journals/ EBCVM/jhome.html
Heart	heart.bmjjournals.com
Journal of the American College of Cardiology	www.cardiosource.com/jacc.html
New England Journal of Medicine	www.nejm.com
The Lancet	www.thelancet.com

Cardiology resources

Cardio.net	www.cardio.net
Cardiology Compass	cardiologycompass.com
Cochrane collaboration	www.cochrane.de
the heart.org	www.theheart.org

Professional organisations

American College of Cardiology	www.acc.org
American Heart Association	www.americanheart.org
British Cardiac Society	www.cardiac.org.uk
British Cardiovascular Intervention Society	www.bcis.org.uk
European Resuscitation Council	www.erc.edu
European Society of Cardiology	www.escardio.org
Royal College of Physicians	www.rcplondon.ac.uk
UK Resuscitation Council	www.resus.org.uk

Guidelines

ACC/AHA practice guidelines	www.acc.org/clinical/guidelines/ index.html
ESC guidelines for patient management	www.escardio/scinfo/guidelines.htm

Trial acronym	Full name	Reference	Authors
4S	Scandinavian Simvastatin Survival Study (4S)	Lancet (1994) 344:1383–1389	Scandinavian Simvastatin Survival Group (4S)
AIRE	Acute Infarction Ramipril Efficacy	Lancet (1993) 342:821–828	The AIRE study investigators
AIREX	AIRE Extension Study	Lancet (1997) 349:1493–1497	Hall AS et al for the AIREX study investigators
ASPIRE	Action on Secondary Prevention through Intervention to Reduce Events	Heart (1996) 75:334-342	Bowker TJ et al
CAMIAT	Canadian Amiodarone Myocardial Infarction Arrhythmia Trial	Lancet (1997) 349:675–682	Cairns JA et al for the CAMIAT investigators
CARE	Cholesterol And Recurrent Events	NEJM (1996) 335:1001–1009	Sacks FM et al for the CARE investigators
CAST	Cardiac Arrhythmia Suppression Trial	NEJM (1991) 324:781–788	Echt DS et al
CONSENSUS II	Cooperative New Scandinavian Enalapril Survival Study II	NEJM (1992) 327:678-684	Swedberg K et al
DAVIT II	Danish Verapamil Infarction Trial II	Am J Cardiol (1990) 66:779–785	The Danish Study Group on Verapamil in Myocardial Infarction
DIGAMI	Diabetes Mellitus, Insulin Glucose Infusion in Acute Myocardial Infarction	BMJ (1997) 314:1512-1515	DIGAMI Study Group

Trial acronym	Full name	Reference	Authors
EAFT	European Atrial Fibrillation Trial	Lancet (1993) 342:1255-1262	European Atrial Fibrillation Trial
EMIAT	European Myocardial Infarction Amiodarone Trial	Lancet (1997) 349:667–674	Julian DG et al for the EMIAT investigators
EPISTENT	Evaluation of Platelet IIb/IIIa Inhibitor for Stenting	Lancet (1998) 352:87-92	The EPISTENT investigators
ESSENCE	Efficacy and Safety of Subcutaneous Enoxaparin in Non-Q-Wave Coronary Events	NEJM (1997) 337:447–452	Cohen M et al
EUROASPIRE	European Action on Secondary Prevention through Intervention to Reduce Events	Eur Heart J. (1997) 18:1569-1582	EUROASPIRE study group
FRIC	Fragmin in Unstable Coronary disease study	Circulation (1996) 96:61–68	Klein W et al
FRISC	Fragmin during Instability in Coronary Artery Disease	Lancet (1996) 347:561–568	FRISC study group
FRISC II	Fragmin during Instability in Coronary Arterial Disease	Lancet (1999) 354:708–715	FRISC II Investigators
GISSI	Gruppo Italiano per lo Studio della Sopravvivenza nell'infarto Miocardico	Lancet (1986) i:397–402	Gruppo Italiano per lo Studio della Streptochinasi nell'infarto Miocardico
GISSI-3	Gruppo Italiano per lo Studio della Sopravvivenza nell'infarto Miocardico	Lancet (1995) 343:1115–1122	Gruppo Italiano per lo Studio della Sopravvivenza nell'infarto Miocardico

Trial acronym	Full name	Reference	Authors
GUSTO	Global Utilisation of Streptokinase and Tissue Plasminogen Activator for Occluded Coronary Arteries	NEJM (1993) 329:673–682	The GUSTO investigators
HOPE	The Heart Outcomes Prevention Evaluation Study	NEJM (2000) 342:145-153	The Heart Outcomes Prevention Evaluation Study Investigators
INJECT	International Joint Efficacy Comparison of Thrombolytics	JACC (1995) 26:1657–1667	Schroder R et al
MIAMI	Metoprolol in Acute Myocardial Infarction	Eur Heart J (1985) 6:199-226	The MIAMI Trial Research Group
ISIS-1	First International Study of Infact Survival	Lancet (1986) ii:57–66	ISIS-1 collaborative group
ISIS-2	Second International Study of Infact Survival	Lancet (1988) ii:349–360	ISIS-2 collaborative group
ISIS-3	Third International Study of Infact Survival	Lancet (1992) 339:753–770	ISIS-3 collaborative group
ISIS-4	Fourth International Study of Infact Survival	Lancet (1995) 345:669–685	ISIS-4 collaborative group
LATE	Late Assessment of Thrombolytic Efficacy	JACC (1996) 27:1327–1332	Langer A et al
MDPIT	Multicenter Diltiazem Postinfarction Trial	NEJM (1988) 319:385–392	The Multicenter Diltiazem Postinfarction Trial Research Group
OASIS	Organisation to Assess Strategies for Ischaemic Syndromes	Lancet (1998) 352:507–514	Yusuf, S et al

Trial acronym	Full name	Reference	Authors
PRAISE	Prospective Randomized Amlodipine Survival Evaluation	NEJM (1996) 335:1107–1114	Prospective Randomized Amlodipine Survival Study Group
SPAF	Stroke Prevention in Atrial Fibrillation	Circulation (1991) 84:527-539	SPAF Investigators
SPAF-II	Stroke Prevention in Atrial Fibrillation II	Lancet (1994) 343:687-691	SPAF Investigators
SPRINT	Secondary Prevention Re-infarction Israeli Nifedipine Trial	Euro Heart J (1988) 9:354–364	The Israeli SPRINT study group
TIMI	Thrombolysis in Myocardial Infarction	Circulation (1987) 76:142–154	Chesebro JH et al
TIMI-IIB	Thrombolysis in Myocardial Infarction	Circulation (1991) 83:422–437	Roberts R et al for TIMI investigators
TRACE	Trandolapril Cardiac Evaluation	NEJM (1995) 333:1670-1676	Kober L et al
VANQWISH	Veterans Affairs Non-Q-Wave Infarction Strategies in Hospital	NEJM (1998) 338:1785–1792	Boden WE et al

ACC	American College of Cardiology
ACE	angiotensin converting enzyme
AF	atrial fibrillation
AHA	American Heart Association
AICD	automatic implantable cardioverter–defibrillator
AMI	acute myocardial infarction
APTT	activated partial thromboplastin time
AV	atrioventricular
BBB	bundle branch block
BCT	broad-complex tachycardia(s)
BD	twice a day
BMI	body mass index
BNF	British National Formulary
BP	blood pressure
BRS	baroreflex sensitivity
CABG	coronary artery by-pass surgery
CAD	coronary artery disease
CCU	Coronary Care Unit
CHB	complete heart block
CK	creatine kinase
CK-MB	MB isoform of creatine kinase
COAD	chronic obstructive airways disease
CPR	cardio-pulmonary resuscitation
CRP	C reactive protein
CVP	central venous pressure
CXR	chest X-ray
DC	direct current
DGH	district general hospital
DVLA	Driver and Vehicle Licensing Authority
ECG	electrocardiogram
GP	general practitioner
GTN	glyceryl trinitrate
HIT	heparin-induced thrombocytopaenia
HMG CoA	hydroxy-methyl-glutarate Coenzyme A
INR	international normalised ratio
IU	international units
IV	intravenous
JVP	jugular venous pressure
LAH	left anterior hemiblock
LBBB	left bundle branch block
LDL	low density lipoprotein
LMWH	low molecular weight heparin

LPH	left posterior hemiblock
LV	left ventricle
LVEF	left ventricular ejection fraction
MET	metabolic equivalent
MI	myocardial infarction
NCT	narrow complex tachycardia
NSAID	non-steroidal anti-inflammatory drug
OD	once a day
PCWP	pulmonary capillary wedge pressure
PO	oral
PRN	as required
PTCA	percutaneous transluminal coronary angioplasty
QDS	four times a day
RBBB	right bundle branch block
RV	right ventricle
RVI	right ventricular infarction
S_aO2	arterial oxygen saturation
SA	sino-atrial
SC	subcutaneous
SCD	sudden cardiac death
SK	streptokinase
TDS	three times a day
TnT	troponin T
tPA	tissue plasminogen activator
U	units
UAP	unstable angina pectoris
UFH	unfractionated heparin
VPB	ventricular premature beat
VSD	ventricular septal defect
VT	ventricular tachycardia
WHO	World Health Organisation

Immediate management of MI

1.1 Immediate management of chest pain compatible with MI

Resuscitate the patient if unstable

If stable
1. Attach ECG and BP monitor
2. Take history and perform examination focusing primarily on the cardiovascular system
3. Obtain a 12 lead ECG (include V_4R and V_7–V_9 in inferior MI to exclude right ventricular and posterior wall involvement)
4. Insert an IV line
5. Take blood, via the IV line if possible, for
     - urea and electrolytes
     - random glucose
     - creatine kinase, troponin or other serum marker of myocardial damage
     - random cholesterol
     - full blood count

The above measures should take no longer than 10–15 min

Proceed to immediate treatment measures (see section 1.2).

Include a brief neurological examination. If thrombolytic treatment is later suspected of causing a stroke (see section 1.8) this will allow determination of whether a neurological deficit is new or old.

V_4R is taken on the right chest in the 'mirror image' position to lead V_4. Right ventricular involvement is indicated with ST elevation of 1 mm or more in lead V_4R.

1.2 Immediate treatment

1. **Give aspirin** 300 mg to chew, then swallow (❂❂❂).
2. **Relieve pain** with diamorphine using 2.5–5 mg aliquots IV (❂❂❂). A total of 10–15 mg, or even more, may be required. Give an anti-emetic, e.g. metoclopramide 10 mg IV with opiates. **Document** the perceived severity of pain on an objective scale before giving opiates or thrombolytic therapy (❂ – see also section 1.7).
3. **Give oxygen** by mask or nasal prongs (❂❂)
4. **Assess for reperfusion therapy** (❂❂❂ – see section 1.3).

Arrange chest X-ray (usually portable). This should not be allowed to delay reperfusion therapy. Do not, for instance, send the patient from the Emergency Department to the CCU via the X-ray Department.

ACC/AHA guidelines also recommend early use of IV nitrates, in patients with large anterior infarctions, congestive heart failure, persistent ischaemia or hypertension (Class I recommendation).

There are few data on the benefits of oxygen use: ACC/AHA recommend routine use if $SaO_2 < 90\%$ (Class I recommendation) and routinely for the first 2–3 h (Class IIa recommendation).

1.3 Definitive treatment

The optimum therapy is to open the infarct-related artery as soon as possible. All patients with a relevant history and appropriate ECG should be given reperfusion therapy or have this option actively rejected.

> If thrombolysis is given aim for a 'door-to-needle' time of less than 30 min (✪✪✪)

Proceed to **immediate** thrombolysis if

1. Consistent history with symptoms <12 h
   AND
2. ECG shows one of the following
   i. ST elevation in at least 2 contiguous leads (✪✪✪) (at least 1 mm in inferior leads; 2 mm in anterior leads)

   ii. Left bundle branch block (✪✪✪ – and see opposite)

   iii. 3 mm or more ST depression in anterior leads (✪ – see section 1.10.1)

   AND
3. No contra-indications to thrombolysis exist (see section 1.4)

> See below and sections 1.4 and 1.5 if MI is suspected but these conditions are not met

Streptokinase is the usual thrombolytic agent used in the UK – see section 1.6 for when to use alternatives.
Streptokinase is given as 1.5 MU over 60 min as an infusion.

tPA is given as a bolus of 15 mg, then infusion of 50 mg over 30 min, then 35 mg over 30 min (max total dose 100 mg).

Following tPA infusion give heparin IV for 48 h to maintain APTT between 2.0 and 3.0. (Some units advise APTT 1.5–2.5.)

There is overwhelming evidence of benefit from reperfusion therapy in patients presenting within the first 24 h after the onset of symptoms. The evidence is strongest for thrombolytic therapy e.g. GISSI, ISIS-2, ISIS-3, GUSTO.

The National Service Framework for Coronary Heart Disease expects 75% of eligible patients to receive thrombolysis within the 30 min target by April 2002 and within 20 min by April 2003.

Reperfusion therapies include

1. **Thrombolytic agent**
   Streptokinase (SK) and tissue plasminogen activator (tPA) are easily the commonest used agents in the UK, although reteplase and anistreplase (APSAC) are also available.
2. **Primary PTCA**
   This option is discussed by e.g. de Belder and Hall[1]. Partly on the basis of their own experience these authors recommend PTCA as primary treatment for MI in the following cases
       i. Patients with a contra-indication to thrombolysis
       ii. Patients presenting with cardiogenic shock
       iii. Patients who re-infarct following thrombolysis
       iv. Patients in whom thrombolysis fails.

Coronary by-pass surgery (CABG) is effectively never used as acute reperfusion therapy in the UK.
The **age** of any LBBB is immaterial to the decision to thrombolyse, although new, or presumed new, LBBB is a strong indicator of acute damage.

In patients <65 kg tPA dose is 15 mg bolus, then 0.75 mg/kg over 30 min, then 0.5 mg/kg over 30 min.

REFERENCE

1. de Belder MA and Hall JA (1999) Infarct angioplasty *Heart* 82:399–401 (✓✓)

7

If history is suggestive of MI but ECGs are not diagnostic

1. Review the history
2. Review ECG to exclude e.g. true posterior MI
3. Repeat ECG e.g. at 10 min intervals for 30 min, then at 30 min intervals until 90 min
4. Await serum markers e.g. CK-MB, Troponin T
5. Exclude aortic dissection

If > 12 h has elapsed since onset of symptoms the benefit of thrombolysis is much smaller, and is likely to be only marginal if 18–24 h have elapsed. Give thrombolysis only if the risk–benefit ratio of treatment is very likely to be in the patient's favour, or if there is clinical or ECG evidence of continuing ischaemia (✪✪✪).

Table 1.1 illustrates the benefits of thrombolysis in certain patient groups, and risks for developing intracranial haemorrhage (ICH) following thrombolysis are also discussed.

Early risk stratification is discussed further in section 2.1. It is possible to identify patients at very high risk (see section 1.10.2 for evidence from MILIS study) and those with very low risks of in-hospital death (see opposite). Risk stratification should aid decision-making when the potential benefit of thrombolytic therapy needs to be weighed carefully against the risks of treatment.

If >24 h has elapsed since symptom onset, there is no evidence of benefit from thrombolytic treatment. Admit the patient to CCU and see section 2.3 for subsequent treatment (✪).

If contra-indications to thrombolytic treatment exist see section 1.5 below.

A 28 day mortality post MI of less than 1% was predicted in a large Australian study for patients who met all the following criteria[2]

  age <60 years
  heart rate <100/min
  typical symptoms at presentation
  no prior MI
  not diabetic
  no significant Q wave in admission ECG

One-third of 6746 patients studied met all of these criteria.

Raised serum markers may confirm myocardial damage. However, there is no evidence that thrombolytic therapy is beneficial in patients with no ECG changes but who do have serum indicators of infarction.

Table 1.1 Benefits of thrombolysis in selected patient groups. Data from reference 3

ECG or patient characteristic at presentation	Lives saved per 1000 patients treated
BBB on presenting ECG	49
Anterior ST elevation	37
Inferior ST elevation	8
Symptom to treatment time <1 h	35
Symptom to treatment time 2–3 h	25
Symptom to treatment time 4–6 h	19
Symptom to treatment time 7–12 h	16
Patients age <55 years	12
Patients aged 65–74 years	26

The relative risks of ICH following thrombolysis are increased in patients who are
>65 years (odds ratio 2.2, 95% CI 1.4–3.5)
<70 kg (odds ratio 2.1, 95% CI 1.3–3.2)
hypertensive on presentation (odds ratio 2.0, 95% CI 1.2–3.2)
treated with tPA (odds ratio 1.6, 95% CI 1.0–2.5)

With 3 of these risk factors present, the absolute risk of ICH is estimated to be between 1.5 and 2.25%[4].

REFERENCES

2. Parsons RW et al (1994) Early identification of patients at low risk of death after myocardial infarction and potentially suitable for early hospital discharge *BMJ* 308:1006–1010 (✓✓)
3. FTT Collaborative Group (1994) Indications for fibrinolytic therapy in suspected myocardial infarction *Lancet* 343:311–322 (✓✓✓)
4. Simmoons ML et al (1993) Individual risk assessment for intracranial haemorrhage during thrombolytic therapy *Lancet* 342: 1523–1528 (✓✓)

1.4 Contra-indications to thrombolytic treatment

Lists of contra-indications are generally based on patho-physiology and clinical experience rather than on trial data. These will therefore differ in different protocols and standard texts. Current European and US recommendations are included below. Significant differences will be noted between these.

Treatment with thrombolytics is generally contra-indicated if the risk of complications outweighs the potential benefit of salvaging myocardium.

Absolute contra-indications

Haemorrhagic stroke at any time (Euro, ACC/AHA)
Other stroke within preceding 12 months (Euro, ACC/AHA)
Known intracranial neoplasm (ACC/AHA)
Active internal bleeding (other than menstrual) (ACC/AHA)
GI bleeding within last month (Euro)
Suspected aortic dissection (Euro, ACC/AHA)
Major surgery within preceding 3 weeks (Euro)

Relative contra-indications

Blood pressure >180/110 at presentation (Euro, ACC/AHA)
History of chronic severe hypertension (ACC/AHA)
Trauma within preceding 2–4 weeks (ACC/AHA)
CPR >10 min, especially with rib fracture (ACC/AHA)
Major surgery within preceding 3 weeks (ACC/AHA)
Intravascular clot e.g. in LA, LV or aortic aneurysm (see reference 6)
Non–compressible vascular puncture (Euro, ACC/AHA)
Active peptic ulcer disease (ACC/AHA)
Pregnancy (Euro, ACC/AHA)
Recent retinal laser treatment (Euro)
Age >75 years, especially female patients (see references 8a and 8b)

Not contra-indications (see opposite)

Proliferative diabetic retinopathy
Warfarin therapy (relative contra–indication in Euro; ACC/AHA)
Menstrual bleeding

Experienced clinicians differ significantly in their management of patients with perceived contra-indications[5].

High blood pressure should be lowered prior to thrombolysis e.g. with beta-blockers or intravenous nitrates.

Recent retrospective analysis from GUSTO has highlighted the excess risk of thrombolysis in those aged over 75[8a,8b].

GUSTO-I showed that proliferative diabetic retinopathy should not be a contra-indication to thrombolytic therapy[7].

Acute MI in the setting of warfarin therapy represents a failure of anti-coagulation and thrombolytic therapy remains appropriate.

Only 12 women in GUSTO-I were menstruating at presentation. 3/12 (25%) had bleeds requiring transfusion compared to 11% of all patients in the GUSTO population. There were no strokes or 'severe' bleeds in menstruating women given tPA[8].

REFERENCES

5. Wald DS (1998) Perceived contraindications to thrombolytic treatment in acute myocardial infarction. A survey at a teaching hospital *J Acc & Emerg Med* 15:329–331 (✓)

6. Stafford PJ et al (1989) Multiple microemboli after disentegration of clot during thrombolysis for acute myocardial infarction *BMJ* 299:1310–1312 (✓)

7. Mahaffey KW et al (1997) Diabetic retinopathy should not be a contraindication to thrombolytic therapy for acute myocardial infarction: review of ocular hemorrhage incidence and location in the GUSTO-I trial *JACC* 30:1606–1610 (✓✓)

8. Karnash SL et al (1995) Treating menstruating women with thrombolytic therapy: insights from the global utilization of streptokinase and tissue plasminogen activator for occluded coronary arteries (GUSTO-I) trial *JACC* 26:1651–1656 (✓✓)

8a. Thiemann DR et al (2000) Lack of benefit for intravenous thrombolysis in patients with myocardial infarction who are older than 75 years *Circulation* 101:2239–2246 (✓✓)

8b. Ayanian JZ, Braunwald E (2000) Thrombolytic therapy for patients with myocardial infarction who are older than 75 years: do the risks outweigh the benefits? *Circulation* 101:2224–2226 (✓✓)

1.5 Management of the patient ineligible for thrombolytic therapy

Patients ineligible for thrombolytic therapy form a high-risk group and may represent more than 30% of patients presenting to UK hospitals with MI[9].

> No patient should be denied reperfusion therapy without the options being actively rejected by someone of appropriate seniority and experience (✪✪✪)

If an absolute contra-indication to thrombolysis exists

Where a large amount of myocardium is in jeopardy, and the patient presents within 12 h of symptoms, contact the local cardiac centre and determine whether primary PTCA or even emergency CABG is feasible (✪✪).

If neither option is possible document the situation and treat using

Aspirin (✪✪✪)
IV heparin if not contra-indicated (✪✪✪)
IV nitrates (✪✪)
Beta-blockers (✪✪✪) The choice of IV or oral use will probably depend on local protocol. See also section 6.2

Magnesium infusion may be beneficial in this group despite the negative data from ISIS-4[10] (✪✪). In LIMIT-2, which did show benefit of using Mg in acute MI, 8 mmol Mg was given IV over 5 min, then 65 mmol was infused over 24 h. In thrombolysed patients the bolus was given before the thrombolytic agent. ACC/AHA suggest 2 g IV over 5–15 min, then 18 g infused over 24 h.

If relative contra-indications exist

1. Assess the clinical risk-benefit ratio of thrombolytic treatment after discussion with senior or specialist colleagues.
2. Document the decision and the basis for it.
3. Treat as above if thrombolysis is not given.

Data from a Nottingham registry indicate that patients who are ineligible for thrombolytic therapy are $>2.6 \times$ (CI 1.6–4.3) more likely to die within 4 years than patients treated with thrombolysis as part of a clinical trial. These latter patients' clinical characteristics differ significantly from non-trial patients[11].

Primary PTCA is where immediate PTCA is used as the means to open the infarct-related artery. In the UK local arrangements will dictate availability of this service. This is currently not widespread, but is likely to increase substantially.

The relative merits of primary PTCA and thrombolysis have been extensively discussed in the literature[12]. See also section 1.3.

Advantages of primary PTCA

1. Better reported TIMI grade 3 flow in the infarct-related vessel (typically >95% for PTCA and 33–50% for thrombolysis) and better overall survival.
2. Very small reported risk of intracranial haemorrhage.
3. Overall cost is probably comparable to thrombolysis.

Disadvantages

1. Needs availability of catheterisation laboratory and suitably experienced staff.
2. Systemic anti-coagulation is still required.

REFERENCES

9. Wong PS et al (1998) The clinical course of patients with acute myocardial infarction who are unsuitable for thrombolytic therapy because of the presenting electrocardiogram *Cor Art Dis* 9:747–752– data from UK Heart Attack Study (✓✓)
10. Woods KL and Fletcher S (1994) Long-term outcome after intravenous magnesium sulphate in suspected acute myocardial infarction: the second Leicester Intravenous Magnesium Intervention Trial (LIMIT-2) *Lancet* 343:816–819; Shechter M et al (1995) Magnesium therapy in acute myocardial infarction when patients are not candidates for thrombolytic therapy *Am J Cardiol* 75:321–323 (✓✓)
11. Brown N et al (1999) Relevance of clinical trial results in myocardial infarction to medical practice: comparison of four year outcome in participants of a thrombolytic trial, patients receiving routine thrombolysis and those deemed ineligible for thrombolysis *Heart* 81:598–602 (✓✓)
12. e.g. in Weaver WD et al (1997) Comparison of primary coronary angioplasty and intravenous thrombolytic therapy for acute myocardial infarction: a quantitative review *JAMA* 278:2110–2111, in *Eur Heart J* (1997) 18:896–899 and in *Heart* editorials (1997) 78:323–328 and (1999) 82:399–404 (✓✓)

1.6 Who should receive tPA?

Many CCUs in the UK have local protocols defining when tPA should be used in preference to streptokinase.

Such policies usually reserve tPA use for 'high-risk' patients such as

> anterior MI
> presenting within 4 h of symptom onset
> previous CABG with vein grafts

Patients who have received SK at any time in the past should also receive tPA, owing to the development of neutralising anti-streptokinase antibodies following prior exposure[13].

Remember that patient factors (Table 2.1) have a far greater influence on outcome than the choice of thrombolytic.

> **It is therefore more important to give treatment quickly than to waste time deciding between treatment options of very similar efficacy (✪✪✪)**

Advantages of tPA

1. Better overall trial survival (10/1000 treatments compared to SK (GUSTO), particularly in high-risk groups. The significance of this apparent advantage has been questioned[14].
2. tPA is non-antigenic so does not stimulate neutralising antibodies and may be used for re-infarction or subsequent MI. tPA confers a survival advantage in patients with previous CABG including vein grafts (GUSTO – see section 1.10.5).

Disadvantages

1. Cost (8–10 × that of streptokinase).
2. Requirement for 48 h heparin post tPA.
3. Higher rate of stroke (3/1000 treatments).

Consensus views

ACC/AHA – 'the cost–benefit ratio is greatest in patients presenting early after onset of chest pain or symptoms and in those with a large area of injury (e.g. anterior infarction) and at low risk of intracranial haemorrhage'.

Euro – 'will depend on an individual assessment of risk and also on factors such as availability and cost benefit'.

Collins R et al (1998)[14] – 'the choice of fibrinolytic regimen appears to make little difference to the overall probability of stroke-free survival, because the regimens that dissolve coronary thrombi more rapidly produce greater risks of cerebral haemorrhage'.

REFERENCES

13. Squire IB et al (1999) Humoral and cellular immune responses up to 7.5 years after administration of streptokinase for acute myocardial infarction *Eur Heart J* 20:1245–1252 (✓✓)
14. Collins R et al (1998) Drug therapy: aspirin, heparin, and fibrinolytic therapy in suspected myocardial infarction *NEJM* 336:847–860 (✓✓✓)

1.7 Assessing reperfusion after thrombolysis

There are three non-invasive methods which have been used to determine the presence or absence of reperfusion of the infarct-related artery following thrombolytic therapy.

1. resolution of chest pain
2. resolution of ST segment elevation
3. biochemical markers

Of these, none is completely satisfactory (see Table 1.2) but ECGs are the most widely used.

Resolution of chest pain

Chest pain is straightforward to quantify on a 1 to 10 scale of severity. Use of such a scale makes it easy to record a patient's response to treatment. However, perception of the pain of MI is very variable and may be affected as much by opiates as by thrombolytic therapy. None the less, several studies have shown this may be a useful predictor of reperfusion in conjunction with others.

Resolution of ST segment elevation

ECG evidence of ST segment recovery toward baseline following thrombolytic therapy provides a useful predictor of prognosis (INJECT). More specifically <50% resolution of ST elevation in the worst lead with no accelerated indoventricular rhythm has been shown to be a useful marker of <TIMI 3 flow in the infarct related artery[16].

Interestingly, ST segment resolution seems to provide a better predictor of outcome than the presence of an open artery at angiography.

Biochemical markers

This is an active area of research. Disappointingly, there is as yet little evidence to show that use of biochemical markers of reperfusion can usefully direct subsequent management. The best currently available approaches are discussed in references 15 and 17.

Table 1.2 Diagnostic utility of non-invasive markers of reperfusion[17]

Marker	Sensitivity	Specificity
Abrupt resolution of chest pain	66–84%	<30%
Resolution of ST segment elevation	52–97%	43–88%
Biochemical marker	CK isoenzymes, troponin T, fatty acid binding proteins and myoglobin have all been used	

'Resolution' was taken by most trials to mean reduction in ST height of 25–50% over all leads showing ST elevation or in the single lead with most ST elevation.

In INJECT, non-resolution of ST elevation was the best predictor of 30 day mortality.

If ST segment resolution was >70%, mortality was 2.5%, this rose to 17.5% if ST segment resolution was <30%.

REFERENCES

15. Christenson RH et al (1997) Assessment of coronary reperfusion after thrombolysis with a model combining myoglobin, creatine kinase-MB, and clinical variables. TAMI-7 Study Group *Circulation* 96:1776–1782 (✓✓✓)

16. Pomes Iparraguirre H et al (1997) Prognostic value of clinical markers of reperfusion in patients with acute myocardial infarction treated by thrombolytic therapy *Am Heart J* 134:631–638 (✓✓✓)

17. Davies CH and Ormerod OJM (1998) Failed coronary thrombolysis *Lancet* 351:1191–1196 (✓✓✓)

RECOMMENDATIONS (largely after data from reference 17)

1. Document patient's perception of pain on an objective scale before and after any thrombolytic therapy (✪).

2. Repeat 12 lead ECG 40 min after thrombolysis, and ideally again 120 min after thrombolysis (✪✪).

3. If pain settles and ST segments resolve assume adequate reperfusion (✪).

4. If ST segments do not resolve in a patient with 5 or fewer involved leads, and patient is haemodynamically stable, assume incomplete reperfusion but take no further action (✪✪).

5. If ST segments do not resolve in a patient with 6 or more involved leads, and patient continues to have pain then repeat thrombolysis or refer for rescue PTCA depending on local availability (✪✪).

6. If ST segments do not resolve in a patient with 6 or more involved leads and patient is haemodynamically stable assume incomplete reperfusion and a large infarct. Discuss with senior or specialist colleagues and repeat thrombolysis or refer for rescue PTCA if the benefits of further treatment are judged to outweigh risk of conservative management (✪).

7. **If patient is haemodynamically unstable, with falling blood pressure and/or increasing heart rate repeat thrombolysis or refer for rescue PTCA whatever the apparent extent of the infarction (✪✪✪).**

'Resolution' was taken by most trials to mean reduction in ST height of 25–50% over all leads with ST elevation or in the single lead with most ST elevation.

The 'number of leads' criterion follows the approach taken by the GISSI investigators and reflects the likely size of infarction.

Some authors recommend rescue PTCA in any case where thrombolysis is thought to have failed[18].

In the rare patient with a large infarct who is haemodynamically stable, evidence is sparse as to the best course of action if initial thrombolysis has failed. Individual cases must therefore be assessed on their merits depending on factors such as the interval between symptoms and treatment, predicted survival (see section 2.2) and pre-morbid condition.

REFERENCE

18. de Belder MA and Hall JA (1999) Infarct angioplasty *Heart* 82:399–401 (✓✓)

1.8 Problems following thrombolytic therapy

Hypotension (usually secondary to streptokinase treatment)

Some fall in BP with streptokinase is virtually inevitable. If the patient is symptomatic stop the infusion. Lay patient flat or head down. Give 250–500 ml of IV colloid if severe. Attempt to re-start thrombolytic if BP improves within 15 min. If less than 50% of the infusion can be completed give tPA instead.

Allergic reaction (almost always secondary to streptokinase)

Stop infusion. Depending on severity give IV hydrocortisone 100 mg and IV chlorpheniramine 10 mg. Give tPA instead.

Headache, unexplained altered conscious level or other symptoms suggestive of haemorrhagic stroke

Stop infusion. Confirm diagnosis, usually via CT scan. Give fresh frozen plasma to normalise clotting, and if heparin is infusing reverse with protamine.

This complication has a high early mortality rate (see opposite) and early discussion with a neurologist may be the best way to determine appropriate levels of intervention.

Other major bleeds

Stop infusion. Definitive treatment such as surgery may be precluded by MI, so usual treatment will be to reverse abnormal clotting with fresh frozen plasma and transfuse blood and fresh platelets as required. If bleeding continues, discuss with surgeon and/or haematologist.

Minor bleeds

If possible achieve haemostasis and continue infusion. Stop thrombolysis only if blood loss is likely to be more dangerous than continuing treatment.

Retrospective analysis from the GUSTO dataset found a 60% 30-day mortality for haemorrhagic stroke in patients suffering this complication following thrombolysis[19].

Predictors of mortality in this study included
> low Glasgow coma scale
> age
> interval between thrombolysis and stroke
> hydrocephalus
> herniation
> mass effect of bleed
> intraventricular extension
> volume of intracranial haemorrhage

REFERENCE

19. Sloan MA et al (1998) Prediction of 30-day mortality among patients with thrombolysis-related intracranial hemorrhage *Circulation* 98:1376–1382 (✓✓)

1.9 Patients with diabetes and acute MI

Patients with acute MI who also have diabetes represent a high-risk group having a 1 year mortality up to twice that of non-diabetics[20].

The DIGAMI trial provided strong evidence that treatment of patients with all types of diabetes, including those controlled on diet alone, is best managed with intravenous insulin in the peri-infarct period[21].

Note too that glucose levels at presentation are a prognostic indicator[21]. It is uncertain if this is because hyperglycaemia is a marker of previous poor control or a metabolic response to the severity of the acute ischaemic insult.

RECOMMENDATIONS

1. **Reperfusion therapy remains the priority of definitive treatment of MI for patients with diabetes (❂❂❂).**
2. Patients presenting with blood glucose levels >11 mmol/l should be treated as diabetic (❂❂❂).
3. All patients with diabetes should have glycaemic control managed with intravenous insulin infusions. Most units will have developed a local protocol. The author's current regimen is listed opposite in Table 1.3. Many patients will require adjustment of such a 'sliding scale' to produce optimal control (❂❂❂).
4. Check serum potassium levels within 1–2 h after starting glucose-insulin infusion since they will fall and may need replacement, possibly intravenously. Some units give glucose-insulin-potassium solutions to minimise this (❂).
5. All patients with diabetes suffering an MI should be referred to a diabetologist prior to discharge for review of their glycaemic control and consideration for long-term insulin treatment (❂❂❂).

Patients with diabetes develop accelerated coronary artery disease (CAD) and are 10 to 20 times over-represented amongst those suffering acute MI[22].

In the DIGAMI trial, diabetic patients with MI were treated acutely with a glucose-insulin infusion, and for at least 1 year with subcutaneous insulin. This strategy showed a reduction from 44% (control) to 33% (insulin treatment) in all-cause mortality during the mean 3.4 year follow-up period. Many UK centres regard the DIGAMI protocol as overly aggressive, producing an unacceptable level of hypoglycaemic episodes.

Table 1.3 Regimen for glucose – insulin infusion
Using 50 units Human Actrapid insulin in 50 ml 0.9% saline, infuse depending on following capillary blood glucose readings

Capillary blood glucose (mmol/l)	Infusion rate (ml/h)
<4	0.5
4.1–7	1
7.1–9	2
9.1–11	3
11.1–17	4
17.1–28	5
>28	6

Proliferative diabetic retinopathy should not be regarded as a contra-indication to thrombolytic therapy[23].

REFERENCES

20. Aronson D et al (1997) Mechanisms determining course and outcome of diabetic patients who have had acute myocardial infarction Ann Intern Med 126:296–306 (✓✓)

21. Malmberg K et al (1999) Glycometabolic state at admission: important risk marker of mortality in conventionally treated patients with diabetes mellitus and acute myocardial infarction *Circulation* 99:2626–2632 (✓✓)

22. Karlson BW et al (1993) Prognosis of acute myocardial infarction in diabetic and non-diabetic patients *Diabetic Medicine* 10:449–454 (✓✓)

23. Mahaffey KW et al (1997) Diabetic retinopathy should not be a contraindication to thrombolytic therapy for acute myocardial infarction: review of ocular hemorrhage incidence and location in the GUSTO-I trial *JACC* 30:1606–1610 (✓✓)

1.10 Treatment of 'difficult' MIs

1.10.1   ST depression on presenting ECG
1.10.2   Cardiogenic shock
1.10.3   'Stuttering' MI
1.10.4   Right ventricular infarction
1.10.5   Previous coronary artery surgery

1.10.1 ST depression on presenting ECG

ST depression occurs in a heterogeneous group of patients with ischaemic chest pain. This type of ECG may present in

1. true posterior MI
2. partial thickness MI
3. unstable angina (diagnosed retrospectively)

Aspirin 300 mg PO should be given to all eligible patients (✪✪✪).
A reasonable, but not validated, strategy would be (✪)

1. repeat clinical assessment
2. check posterior chest leads i.e. V_7–V_9
3. repeat ECG 30 and 60 min after first trace

RECOMMENDATIONS

1. **Give thrombolysis if all the following conditions are satisfied (✪)**
   If good clinical evidence of MI exists
   AND
   there is ECG evidence of acute posterior MI
   or there is 3 mm ST depression
   AND
   no possibility exists for primary PTCA.
2. Otherwise, treat as for unstable angina (✪✪ – see section 5.1).

Subgroups with ST depression who might benefit from thrombolysis have not been defined (ACC/AHA). ISIS-2 data suggested a detrimental effect of thrombolysis, but the confidence intervals were wide and a beneficial effect could not be excluded[24]. The LATE study suggests this group might indeed derive some benefit from thrombolysis. Thrombolysis is probably appropriate in true posterior infarction (where ST depression may be confined to V_1–V_4).

ST depression becomes a good discriminator as it becomes deeper and appears in more leads. If it exceeds 3 mm the specificity for MI is 90% (i.e. similar to ST elevation). Moreover, the depth of ST depression is related to subsequent mortality[25].

REFERENCES

24. Rawles J (1997) Should patients with suspected acute myocardial infarction without ST elevation be given thrombolytic treatment? *Eur Heart J* 18:899–906 (✓✓)
25. Lee HS et al (1993) Patients with suspected myocardial infarction who present with ST depression *Lancet* 342:1204–1207 (✓✓)

1.10.2 Cardiogenic shock

This can be defined as systolic BP <90 mmHg for >60 min with evidence of vital organ hypoperfusion e.g. confusion or oliguria. Cardiogenic shock complicates about 7% of all infacts, and this proportion has remained remarkably constant over many years, in both North America and Europe[26,27].

The most important consideration is to open the occluded infarct-related artery, although the best way to achieve this is unclear.

Exclude and/or treat potentially reversible causes such as
> hypovolaemia
> right ventricular MI
> vasovagal reactions
> electrolyte disturbances
> drug side-effects
> arrhythmias
> cardiac tamponade

RECOMMENDATIONS

i Give reperfusion therapy wherever possible (✪✪✪)

If initial thrombolysis has failed to secure reperfusion (see section 1.7) give or repeat tPA if the patient is still a candidate for thrombolysis. Observational studies suggest salvage PTCA is more successful than medical therapy[28]. If local arrangements allow, contact local cardiac centre to see if salvage PTCA is feasible.

ii Optimise monitoring (✪✪)

Swan–Ganz pulmonary artery catheterisation, and intra-arterial BP monitoring will allow the best management of fluid replacement and inotrope therapy.
Insert urinary catheter for hourly urine measurement.

iii Optimise haemodynamics (✪✪)

Correct acidosis, which is almost invariable. Catecholamines work poorly in an acid milieu.
Aim for pulmonary capillary wedge pressure (PCWP) of 15–18 mmHg, and cardiac index of >2 l/min (Euro). Cardiac index is the cardiac output divided by the body surface area (BSA).

Table 1.4 suggests treatments depending on the haemodynamic picture revealed by invasive monitoring. These recommendations are from the 'pre-thrombolytic' era, but are pathophysiologically sound.

Cardiogenic shock carries a mortality of at least 55–80% even in clinical trial populations. Enlist senior and/or specialist help early.

In the MILIS study, cardiogenic shock was found in 7.1% of 845 patients with MI, with a 65% in-hospital mortality. Five independent predictors of developing shock post MI were found
> age >65 years
> admission LV ejection fraction <35%
> peak CK-MB > 160 IU/l
> diabetes
> prior myocardial infarction

With 3, 4 and 5 risk factors present the chances of developing cardiogenic shock were 17.9%, 33.7% and 54.4% respectively[29].

Table 1.4 Treatments in cardiogenic shock depending on haemodynamic picture[30]

	Normal BP	Low BP
Increased PCWP	Diuretic and vasodilator	Diuretic and inotrope ± vasodilator
Low PCWP	Volume expansion	Volume expansion ± inotrope

REFERENCES

26. Goldberg RJ et al (1999) Temporal trends in cardiogenic shock complicating acute myocardial infarction *NEJM* 340:1162–1168 (✓)
27. Danchin N et al (1997) Management of acute myocardial infarction in intensive care units in 1995: a nationwide French survey of practice and early hospital results *JACC* 30: 1598–1605 (✓)
28. Berger PB et al (1997) Impact of an aggressive invasive catheterization and revascularization strategy on mortality in patients with cardiogenic shock in the GUSTO-I trial. An observational study *Circulation* 96:122–127 (✓)
29. Hands ME et al (1989) The in-hospital development of cardiogenic shock after myocardial infarction: incidence, predictors of occurrence, outcome and prognostic factors. The MILIS Study Group *JACC* 14:40–46 (✓✓)
30. Crexells C et al (1973) Optimal level of filling pressure in the left side of the heart in acute myocardial infarction *NEJM* 289:1263–1266 (✓✓)

iv Start inotrope and other supportive therapy (✪✪– Euro)

Relieve pain promptly.
Aim to keep oxygen saturations >97%.

If BP <80 mmHg use noradrenaline (norepinephrine) 2–20 µg/min.

If BP 80–90 mmHg add dopamine 5–15 µg/kg/min and wean noradrenaline (norepinephrine).

If BP rises to >90 mmHg add dobutamine and reduce dopamine to a maximum of 5µg/kg/min.

If there is no response to catecholamine infusion, or they provoke arrhythmias or ischaemic pain secondary to tachycardias, milrinone (or another phosphodiesterase inhibitor such as enoximone) is a possible alternative. Usual dose range for milrinone is 0.25–0.75 µg/kg/min.

If expertise is available, ACC/AHA recommend that an intra-aortic balloon pump be inserted if PTCA or CABG is planned.

1.10.3 'Stuttering' MI

This refers to patients who have recurrent episodes of myocardial ischaemia (or infarction as judged by serum markers) without ECG changes diagnostic of MI.
They should be treated as for unstable angina (see section 5.1), and referred for consideration of in-patient coronary angiography (Class I ACC/AHA recommendation – ✪✪✪).

Despite these recommendations there is no good prospective evidence that noradrenaline (norepinephrine) improves outlook in cardiogenic shock. Many UK authorities avoid using noradrenaline (norepinephrine), since there is little or no evidence it improves either the overall haemodynamic picture or outcome.

1.10.4 Right ventricular infarction

Diagnosis

The combination of hypotension, raised JVP and clear lung fields is a specific but insensitive indicator of RV infarction occurring in fewer than 10% of patients with inferior MI.

The best ECG indicator of RV involvement is ST elevation in lead V_4R. This may persist only up until 24–48 h post MI. ST elevation in V_1 and V_2 in the presence of inferior MI may also indicate RV involvement.

> RV infarction may manifest as cardiogenic shock

RECOMMENDATIONS

i. Maintain right ventricular preload (✪✪)

Keep the patient well hydrated, preferably with oral fluids. If the JVP is low the patient is almost certainly under-hydrated. Avoid, as far as possible, diuretic and nitrate therapy. Note these are commonly used in treating isolated left heart failure. ACE inhibitors and opioid treatment may also contribute to RV pre-load reduction.

ii. Use invasive haemodynamic monitoring in sicker patients (✪✪)

A multi-lumen pulmonary artery (Swan–Ganz) catheter is recommended, since this gives information about both right and left sided filling pressures. Optimal left atrial filling pressure is usually 15–20 mmHg[31]. Right atrial pressures may need to be kept to at least 10–20 mmHg to optimise RV performance.

Left atrial filling pressures are equivalent to pulmonary capillary wedge (PCW) pressures, and right atrial pressures can be measured directly as the central venous pressure (CVP).

iii. Use volume loading or inotropes if required haemodynamically (✪✪)

Judicious volume loading may dramatically improve cardiac output, particularly if diuretics or vasodilators have been used. A reasonable regimen is to assess the response to 200 ml 0.9% saline, and infuse 1000–2000 ml over the next 1–2 h, depending on haemodynamic response and filling pressures. If filling pressures are adequate and the low output state persists dobutamine (usually 5–10 μg/kg/min) should be commenced, and the patient treated as for cardiogenic shock (section 1.10.2).

If ECG evidence of right ventricular infarction exists in inferior MI this is predictive of a worse prognosis (Zehender M et al (1993) *NEJM* 328:981–988). This may be because ST elevation of >1 mV (i.e. >1 mm) in lead V_4R is associated with a larger infarct size rather than because RV involvement is an independent indicator of bad prognosis[32].

Right ventricular infarction increased in-hospital mortality from 6% to 22% in one series of almost 800 patients, although this effect was largely confined to elderly patients[33].

The overall incidence of right ventricular infarction in patients with inferior MI was 32–37% in the above two studies.

REFERENCES

31. Forrester JS (1976) Medical therapy of acute myocardial infarction by application of haemodynamic subsets *NEJM* 295:1356–1362 (✓✓)
32. Zeymer U et al (1998) Effects of thrombolytic therapy in acute inferior myocardial infarction with or without right ventricular involvement *JACC* 32:876–881 (✓✓)
33. Bueno H et al (1998) Combined effect of age and right ventricular involvement on acute inferior myocardial infarction prognosis *Circulation* 98:1714–1720 (✓✓)

Patients with significant RV dysfunction deteriorate significantly if they develop atrial fibrillation or AV block. AF should be treated promptly, either with DC cardioversion or anti-arrhythmics. AV block should be paced. The ideal is to use AV sequential pacing, but since this is rarely possible outside cardiothoracic surgical units in the UK, right ventricular pacing is more usual.

1.10.5 Previous coronary surgery using vein grafts

Where an acute MI is presumed to be due to occlusion of vein grafts, tPA appears to be superior to streptokinase as a thrombolytic agent.
(❂❂❂ – GUSTO 30 day mortality: 8.3% vs 11%).

Subsequent CCU management of MI

2.1 Early CCU management – day 0

Once the patient is on CCU, complete the history and examination with particular respect to
> haemodynamics
> presence of left or right heart failure
> oxygenation
> neurological function

Assess the response to
> pain relief
> reperfusion therapy (see section 1.7)

Review blood results and chest X-ray
Aim for serum K^+ of at least 4.0 mmol/l, and preferably 4.5 or over. Give oral K^+ supplements if K^+ is 3.5–4.0 mmol/l, and re-check K^+ within 4–6 h. If K^+ <3.5 give 10 mmol KCl intravenously over 1 h e.g. in 250 ml 5% dextrose, and re-check following infusion.

Severe potassium depletion is often associated with magnesium depletion so give magnesium if IV potassium replacement is required (e.g. as 5 g $MgSO_4$ in 0.9% NaCl over 1 h, followed by a further 5 g over 24 h).

Administer beta-blocker (✪✪✪) if there is evidence of high adrenergic drive e.g. heart rate >100, systolic BP >160 mmHg. Local protocols may determine use of intravenous rather than oral route for first dose (see section 6.2).

Perform early risk stratification (✪✪✪ – see section 2.2)

There is a clear relationship between hypokalaemia and the frequency of VF in acute MI. In a study of 1074 patients with acute MI, VF was found in 17.2% of patients with serum K^+ <3.6 mmol/l, but in only 7.4% of patients with serum K^+ above this level[34].

REFERENCE

34. Nordrehaug JE and von der Lippe G (1983) Hypokalaemia and ventricular fibrillation in acute myocardial infarction *Brit Heart J* 50:525–529 (✓✓)

2.2 Early risk stratification

Consideration of straightforward clinical data allows early risk stratification using e.g. the Killip classification[35], see Table 2.2. Useful and simple clinical models have been derived from admission clinical variables[36]. More detailed models are available, with well-validated predictive value[37]. The GUSTO based estimates are tedious to calculate manually but are easily dealt with by a simple spreadsheet program.

Risk stratification at this stage is useful in identifying high-risk patients, who will need senior and/or specialist involvement, and low-risk patients who can be discharged early from CCU.

Note that clinical factors have far more influence on survival than differences between thrombolytic regiments, see Table 2.1. The first 5 factors account for almost 90% of 30 day mortality.

2.2.1 Identification of low-risk patients

Patients with 28 day mortality of <1% can be identified post MI. In a large Australian study ($n = 6746$), patients who met all the following criteria

> age <60 years
> heart rate <100/min
> typical symptoms at presentation
> no prior MI
> not diabetic
> no significant Q wave in **admission** ECG

had 28 day mortality at this level. One-third of patients studied met these criteria.

Since the risk of fatal stroke with thrombolytic therapy may exceed this level there is an argument for not using thrombolysis in patients with very low predicted mortality (Thompson).

Table 2.1 Factors predicting early mortality post MI[37]

Factor	Proportion of 30 day risk (%)
Age	31
Systolic BP	24
Killip class	15
Heart rate	12
Location of MI	6
Prior MI	2.8
Hypertension, diabetes, smoking	2.5
Height, weight	1.8
Prior cardiovascular disease or CABG	1.2
Time to treatment	1
tPA vs SK as thrombolytic	0.8

REFERENCES

35. Killip T and Kimball JT (1967) Treatment of myocardial infarction in a coronary care unit. A two year experience with 250 patients *Am J Cardiol* 20:457–464 (✓)
36. e.g. Hillis LD et al (1990) Risk stratification before thrombolytic therapy in patients with acute myocardial infarction *JACC* 16:313–315; Normand ST et al (1996). Using admission characteristics to predict short-term mortality from myocardial infarction in elderly patients. Results from the Cooperative Cardiovascular Project *JAMA* 275:1322–1328 (✓✓)
37. Jacobs DR Jr et al (1999) PREDICT: A simple risk score for clinical severity and long-term prognosis after hospitalization for acute myocardial infarction or unstable angina: the Minnesota heart survey *Circulation* 100:599–607; Lee KL et al (1995) Predictors of 30-day mortality in the era of reperfusion for acute myocardial infarction. Results from an international trial of 41,021 patients. GUSTO-I Investigators *Circulation* 91:1659–1668 (✓✓✓)
38. Parsons RW et al (1994) Early identification of patients at low risk of death after myocardial infarction and potentially suitable for early hospital discharge *BMJ* 308:1006–1010 (✓✓)

2.2.2 Identification of high-risk patients

In the MILIS study, five independent predictors of developing cardiogenic shock post MI were found

age >65 years
admission LV ejection fraction <35%
peak CK–MB >160 IU/l
diabetes
prior myocardial infarction

With 3, 4 and 5 risk factors present the chances of developing cardiogenic shock were 17.9%, 33.7% and 54.4% respectively[39].

RECOMMENDATIONS

1. Perform and document an estimate of clinical outcome based on e.g. Killip classification and above data (✪✪✪).
2. Seek senior or specialist advice if the patient is at significant risk of developing cardiogenic shock (✪✪ – see section 1.10.2).

Table 2.2 Killip class and clinical outcome in 1967[35] and in 1993 (GUSTO)

Killip class	Clinical features of cardiac failre	In-hospital mortality in 1967[35] (%)	GUSTO 30 day mortality (%)
I	No failure	6	5
II	Mild to moderate;S3, crackles in <50% lungs	17	14
III	Severe; S3 and crackles in >50% lungs	38	32
IV	Cardiogenic shock	81	58

REFERENCE

39. Hands ME et al (1989) The in-hospital development of cardiogenic shock after myocardial infarction: incidence, predictors of occurrence, outcome and prognostic factors. The MILIS Study Group *JACC* 14:40–46 (✓✓)

2.3 Patient assessment – day 1 onwards post MI

Post MI patients on CCU need examining at least daily to assess their haemodynamic status and response to therapy, and to plan the next stage of management.

This requires a minimum assessment of

> heart rate and rhythm
> heart and chest auscultation
> JVP or CVP
> blood pressure
> peripheral perfusion

Review that day's ECG and available blood results.

Review medication, and patient's suitability for

> aspirin
> beta–blocker
> ACE inhibitor
> statin (HMG Co-A reductase inhibitor)
> insulin

Ensure the patient is aware of their diagnosis, how they have been treated, and their likely subsequent hospital course.

Review modifiable risk factors with the patient, e.g. smoking, blood pressure, cholesterol, diabetic control, weight and exercise. There will be no better opportunity to persuade a smoker to give up!

In uncomplicated cases patients should be fit for discharge from CCU at about 48 h post MI and for discharge home at 5–7 days.

Further information on specific drugs is given in section 6.

2.4 Complications of MI

2.4.1 Acute pulmonary oedema

Immediate management is similar to the non-MI patient (✪✪)
>   Sit up, give oxygen
>   IV loop diuretic e.g. furosemide (frusemide) 20–40 mg initially
>   IV diamorphine 2.5–5 mg plus IV anti-emetic
>   IV nitrate infusion, titrating to keep systolic BP >100 mmHg
>   Commence oral ACE inhibitor

Check for, and correct if possible
>   electrolyte disturbance, including Ca and Mg
>   recurrent myocardial ischaemia (see sections 2.4.3–4)
>   arrhythmias (see section 2.4.2)
>   hypertension
>   new MR or VSD (see sections 2.4.6–7)
>   infection

Profound anxiety is common in the patient, and sometimes in the medical attendant! There is little to be gained by hovering around the bed. Treat the patient and review in 15–30 min (✪).

Definitive management will be directed at the perceived underlying cause, particularly if there is a new mechanical defect such as papillary muscle rupture or VSD (see e.g. sections 2.4.6 and 2.4.7). If none is apparent, continue supportive treatment, ensuring good oxygenation and pain relief (✪).

If the patient does not respond to the above measures discuss with senior or specialist colleagues the patient's suitability for mechanical ventilation and/or intra-aortic balloon pumping (✪).

Patients in acute pulmonary oedema often tolerate high doses of IV nitrates well. Glyceryl trinitrate has a short half-life and rapid infusion of 100–150 µg may be very effective.

2.4.2 Arrhythmias

2.4.2.1 Tachycardias

  i. Atrial fibrillation
  ii. Ventricular tachycardia
  iii. Ventricular fibrillation
  iv. Atrial premature beats
  v. Ventricular premature beats
  vi. Idioventricular rhythm

i. Atrial fibrillation

This occurs in 10–15% of patients post MI and predicts an adverse prognosis with increased rates of in-hospital death and stroke[40].

AF has different clinical characteristics depending on the site of infarction – see Table 2.3 opposite. In many cases it will revert spontaneously within 12–24 h.

Treatment aims:
1. Immediate DC cardioversion of haemodynamically unstable patient
2. Conversion to sinus rhythm
3. Ventricular rate control
4. Prevention of embolic complications
5. Prevention of recurrence

Table 2.3 Characteristics of AF depending on site of MI

Anterior MI	Inferior MI
Usually occurs after >24 h	Often occurs early
Minimal preceding atrial ectopic activity	Frequent associated atrial ectopic activity, atrial flutter, or atrial tachycardia
Fast ventricular response with haemodynamic compromise	Often does not have fast ventricular response
Often responds well to heart rate slowing and anti-arrhythmics	Frequently resistant to anti-arrhythmics

REFERENCE

40. Crenshaw BS et al (1997) Atrial fibrillation in the setting of acute myocardial infarction: the GUSTO-I experience *JACC* 30:406–413

RECOMMENDATIONS

1. DC cardiovert any haemodynamically unstable patient (✪✪✪ – e.g. altered conscious level, BP<90 mmHg, refractory angina).
2. Heparinise. Aim for APTT 2.0–3.0 (✪✪).
3. Establish ventricular rate control (✪ – see Table 2.4).

Cardioversion is **not** a preferred acute option in the **uncompromised** patient since the substrate for AF is often persistent, making recurrences relatively common (Thompson).

Preferred agents for prevention of recurrence include sotalol and amiodarone (Euro, ACC/AHA).

Once the patient has stabilised DC cardioversion can be attempted as a pre-discharge measure if the patient is kept on heparin. Alternatively the patient can be orally anticoagulated and cardioversion attempted at 4–6 weeks post MI.

Table 2.4 Agents of use in controlling post MI AF

IV beta-blocker **Sotalol** 40–120 mg in 40 mg aliquots **Atenolol** 2.5–5 mg over 5 min to total of 10 mg in 10–15 min **Metoprolol** 2.5–5 mg over 5 min to total of 10 mg in 10–15 min **Esmolol**	*Advantages* Rapid response May convert to SR, particularly if AF secondary to ischaemia Esmolol has a very short half-life of around 9 min *Disadvantages* Negatively inotropic (only limited problem with esmolol)
IV digoxin 0.5 mg over 30 min Repeat in 2–4 h	*Advantages* Reasonably rapid response (30–120 min) Positively inotropic *Disadvantages* May be no better than placebo at converting patient to SR
IV amiodarone 300 mg over 1 h 900 mg over 24 h	*Advantages* No significant negative inotropy Frequent conversion to SR *Disadvantages* Requires central line or 'long line' for administration May require additional agent such as digoxin to achieve adequate rate control
IV verapamil 1–2 mg slow bolus Repeat to max of 10 mg	*Advantages* Rapid effect *Disadvantages* Significant negative inotropy Potentially dangerous when given with beta-blocker

ii. Ventricular tachycardia

Ensure K^+ >4.0 and Mg^{2+} >1.0 mmol/l.

> VT occurring more than 12 h post MI should be discussed with a specialist centre as coronary angiography and invasive electrophysiological assessment may be warranted

The following recommendations give priority to European Resuscitation Council Guidelines.

(conscious patients require general anaesthetic before DC shock)

1. *Sustained polymorphic VT (>30 s or causing haemodynamic collapse)*
   Treat as for VF, i.e. unsynchronised DC shock
   200 J then 200 J, then 360 J

2. *Sustained monomorphic VT with haemodynamic compromise*
   Synchronised DC shock 100 J then 200 J then 360 J

3. *'Torsades de pointes' VT with long QT interval*
   Use bolus Mg 1–2 g IV over 5 min
   (Class IIa ACC/AHA)

4. *Tolerated monomorphic VT*
   Several treatment options exist
   IV sotalol 40–160 mg in slow 40 mg boluses

ACC/AHA recommendations for haemodynamically tolerated VT

a. IV lidocaine (lignocaine) 1–1.5 mg/kg bolus (max 100 mg). If required, give supplemental boluses of 0.5 to 0.75 mg/kg every 5 to 10 min to a maximum of 3 mg/kg total followed by infusion 2–4 mg/min (see BNF).

b. IV procainamide 20–30 mg/min to maximum of 12–17 mg/kg. This may be followed by an infusion of 1 to 4 mg/min. Maximum acute dose 1 g. Use lower infusion rates if renal function abnormal.

c. IV amiodarone 150 mg over 10 min, followed by 1 mg/min for 6 h, then maintenance of 0.5 mg/min.

Overdrive ventricular pacing is also effective and avoids the disadvantages of anti-arrhythmic drugs (see section 7.1.2).

Serum magnesium levels are a poor reflection of tissue magnesium levels, which may be more important pathophysiologically. It may be easier to replace magnesium empirically, which is safe, (e.g. as 5 g $MgSO_4$ in 0.9% NaCl over 1 h, followed by a further 5 g over 24 h) than to have to wait for a serum level which may offer a false sense of security.

Non-sustained VT predicts increased mortality post MI when it occurs 13 h from presentation, the relative risk increasing to a plateau at approximately 24 h post-presentation[41].

Sotalol may be more effective at terminating VT than is lidocaine (lignocaine)[42].

REFERENCES

41. Cheema AN et al (1998) Nonsustained ventricular tachycardia in the setting of acute myocardial infarction *Circulation* 98:2030–2036 (✓✓)
42. Ho DS et al (1994) Double-blind trial of lignocaine versus sotalol for acute termination of spontaneous sustained ventricular tachycardia *Lancet* 344:18–23 (✓✓✓)

5. *'VT storm' i.e. drug-resistant/recurrent VT*

   VT storm is always difficult to control. It is often a consequence of myocardial ischaemia and increased sympathetic outflow. Try (✪)

   IV beta-blockade

   IV amiodarone

If the patient does not settle contact a specialist centre for transfer. Further potential treatments include intra-aortic balloon pumping and emergency revascularisation.

> **The need for continued anti-arrhythmic therapy (particularly infusions) should be reviewed after 6–24 h**

iii. Ventricular fibrillation

Ensure K^+ >4.0 mmol/l and Mg^{2+} >1.0 mmol/l (✪✪).

VF occurring more than 24 h post MI should be discussed
with a specialist centre as further electrophysiological
assessment may be warranted

**The following recommendations give priority to European
Resuscitation Council Guidelines**

Unsynchronised DC shock

> **200 J**
> **then 200 J**
> **then 360 J**

Give CPR for 1 min
Repeat defibrillation at 360 J ×3 within 1 min
Repeat cycle
Give adrenaline (epinephrine) every 3 min
Adjunctive treatment if unsuccessful

1. IV lidocaine (lignocaine) 1.5 mg/kg
2. IV bretylium 5–10 mg/kg
3. IV amiodarone 150 mg bolus

The need for continued anti-arrhythmic therapy
(particularly infusions) should be reviewed after 6–24 h

There is a clear relationship between hypokalaemia and the frequency of VF in acute MI[43]. Increased sympathetic activation in the peri-infarct period is one mechanism why serum potassium levels may be low or low normal.

Serum magnesium levels are a poor reflection of tissue magnesium levels, which may be more important pathophysiologically. It may be easier to replace magnesium empirically, which is safe, (e.g. as 5 g $MgSO_4$ in 0.9% NaCl over 1 h, followed by a further 5 g over 24 h), than to have to wait for a serum level which may offer a false sense of security.

REFERENCE

43. Nordrehaug JE and von der Lippe G (1983) Hypokalaemia and ventricular fibrillation in acute myocardial infarction *Brit Heart J* 50:525–529 (✓✓)

iv. Atrial premature beats
No therapy required.

v. Ventricular premature beats
VPBs are an invariable finding in the immediate post-MI period, with no prognostic significance (Thompson).

There is no evidence that attempting to prevent VPBs is beneficial. Agents such as flecainide have proved actively detrimental in this context (CAST).

No specific therapy is required (✪✪). Correct electrolytes, and treat only symptomatic, non-sustained VT as above.

vi Idioventricular rhythm 'Slow VT'
Frequently seen in acute MI, and regarded by many as a marker of reperfusion following thrombolysis. This rhythm occurs when an ectopic ventricular focus discharges faster than the sinus node.

Idioventricular rhythm usually resolves within 12–24 h. Treatment is unlikely to be required and is recommended only if symptomatic hypotension results.

If treatment is required, the possibilities include (✪)
1. Augment SA nodal rate (e.g. with IV atropine 0.6 mg)
2. Atrial pacing (or ventricular pacing if this is not possible)

2.4.2.2 Bradycardias (Heart rate <50/min)

> Most bradycardias causing symptoms will require treatment
> with atropine or with pacing

i.   Sinus bradycardia
ii. Hemiblock and bundle branch block (BBB)
iii. Atrioventricular (AV) block

i. Sinus bradycardia

Requires no treatment if asymptomatic. Use atropine 0.6 mg IV if associated with low BP, ischaemia or ventricular escape arrhythmias
Reduce dose of beta-blocker or other rate-slowing agent, or stop them altogether.

ii. Hemiblock and bundle branch block (BBB)

Neither left anterior hemiblock (LAH) or left posterior hemiblock (LPH) is independently associated with adverse prognosis but
LAH suggests extensive anterior MI.
LAH requires pacing if associated with RBBB (see below).

iii. Atrioventricular (AV) block

> The consequences of AV block usually depend on whether
> the infarction has predominantly affected anterior or
> inferior territory

With any degree of AV block, AV nodal blocker agents (beta-blockers, diltiazem, verapamil, digoxin) should be avoided wherever possible.

a. first degree (✪✪)
Inferior MI: benign, no treatment required.

Anterior MI: indicates extensive damage involving the interventricular septum. No active treatment is required.

b. second degree – Mobitz type I, Wenckebach (✪✪)
Inferior MI: occurs secondary to AV node ischaemia and is generally benign and self-limiting.

Anterior MI: seen only rarely and usually then with BBB which has more potential for bradycardic complications.

c. second degree – Mobitz type II (✪✪✪)
Inferior MI: seen only rarely. Treat only if symptomatic.

Anterior MI: seen in large infarcts with involvement of the septal conduction system. May progress unpredictably to CHB with sudden clinical deterioration. Transvenous or standby external pacing is therefore required (Thompson; ACC/AHA).

d. complete (third degree)
Inferior MI: CHB may be surprisingly well tolerated and there is often an adequate ventricular rate. Pacing is only recommended with symptomatic bradycardia or haemodynamic compromise unresponsive to atropine (✪✪).

Anterior MI: there is almost always extensive anterior and septal infarction. Transvenous or standby external pacing is required, and the patient is likely to require permanent pacing (✪✪✪).

RECOMMENDATIONS for temporary transvenous pacing
(Class 1 ACC/AHA – ✪✪✪)

1. Asystole.
2. Symptomatic bradycardia of any origin (includes sinus bradycardia with hypotension and Mobitz type I second-degree block unresponsive to atropine).
3. Bilateral BBB of any age (alternating LBBB/RBBB or RBBB with alternating LAH/LPH).
4. New or indeterminate age bifascicular block (RBBB with LAH or LPH, or LBBB) with first-degree AV block.
5. Mobitz type II second-degree AV block.

ACC/AHA recommend that transcutaneous pacing be tried in the following cases

1. Sinus bradycardia (<50 bpm) with symptoms of hypotension (systolic BP<80 mmHg) unresponsive to drug therapy.
2. Mobitz type II second-degree AV block.
3. Third-degree heart block.
4. Bilateral BBB of any age.
5. New or indeterminate age LBBB, LBBB and LAH, RBBB and LPH.
6. RBBB or LBBB and first-degree AV block.

RECOMMENDATIONS for atropine (Class 1 ACC/AHA – ✪✪✪)

1. Symptomatic sinus bradycardia (i.e. HR <50 associated with hypotension, ischaemia or escape ventricular arrhythmias).
2. Asystole.
3. Symptomatic AV block occurring at AV nodal level (Mobitz type I or CHB with narrow-complex escape).

Sections 2.4.3–2.4.5 Chest pain post MI

2.4.3 Re-infarction

In-hospital re-infarction is rare in patients who have received both thrombolysis and aspirin, with an average incidence of 3–4% (ACC/AHA). Re-infarction should be suspected with recurrent ischaemic pain lasting >20 min occurring with ST segment elevation and/or CK or Troponin elevation to >150% of the previous value.

Treatment should be as for failed primary thrombolysis (see section 1.7). If further thrombolysis is planned tPA should be used rather than streptokinase.

2.4.4 Post-MI angina

Recurrent ischaemic pain following thrombolytic therapy is surprisingly common, being reported in up to 58% of patients in one series[44]. Chest pain is likely to be ischaemic if it is similar to presenting symptoms, occurs at rest or occurs on early mobilisation. It may be associated with ST segment or T wave changes on the ECG, or with a further rise in markers of myocardial damage.

RECOMMENDATIONS

1. Perform an ECG during any episode of post MI pain which is likely to be ischaemic in origin (✪✪✪).
2. Take blood for CK, Troponin or other marker of myocardial damage (✪).
3. Treat as for unstable angina (✪✪ – see section 5.1).
4. If not able to mobilise following treatment refer for early coronary angiography (✪✪).

REFERENCE

44. Schaer DH et al (1987) Recurrent early ischemic events after thrombolysis for acute myocardial infarction *Am J Cardiol* 59: 788–792 (✓)

2.4.5 Pericarditis

It is important to distinguish pericarditic pain from recurrent myocardial ischaemia. The history will usually be helpful. Pericarditis is unlikely in the first 24 h post MI. Further indicators of pericarditis include a positional or inspiratory component to the pain or radiation to the left shoulder or scapula. An audible rub is diagnostic, especially if the patient is lying flat. A pericardial rub is heard in 10–15% of patients post MI (Thompson).

ECG findings suggestive of pericarditis in this setting include J point elevation with concave upward ST segment elevation and PR depression (ACC/AHA).

Treatment is with aspirin PO 150–300 mg/day but high doses such as 600 mg 4–6 hourly may be required. Non-steroidal anti-inflammatory agents e.g. indometacin 50 mg PO also offer good symptomatic relief. There is a theoretical objection to their use in that they may cause increased coronary vascular tone and predispose to thinning of the developing myocardial scar (ACC/AHA). In practice this is unlikely to be a problem, especially if only one or two doses are required. Patients experiencing concomitant nausea or vomiting can be treated with indometacin suppositiories.

Echocardiography is not generally useful in managing pericarditis since significant effusion is seen in only 40% of patients with a rub and small effusions can be seen in the majority of post MI patients[45].

Echocardiography remains useful if there is clinical suspicion of cardiac tamponade.

While pericarditis itself is usually benign and self-limiting it may be a marker of a relatively large infarct. Overall, patients with pericarditis have lower ejection fractions and a higher subsequent incidence of heart failure[46,47].

REFERENCES

45. Cheitlin MD et al (1997) ACC/AHA Guidelines for the Clinical Application of Echocardiography. A report of the American College of Cardiology/American Heart Association Task Force on Practice Guidelines (Committee on Clinical Application of Echocardiography). Developed in collaboration with the American Society of Echocardiography. *Circulation* 95:1686–1744 (✓✓✓)
46. Tofler GH et al (1989) Pericarditis in acute myocardial infarction: characterization and clinical significance *Am Heart J* 117:86–92 (✓✓✓)
47. Wall TC et al (1990) Usefulness of a pericardial friction rub after thrombolytic therapy during acute myocardial infarction in predicting amount of myocardial damage. The TAMI Study Group *Am J Cardiol* 66:1418–1421 (✓✓)

Sections 2.4.6–2.4.8
Mechanical complications post MI

2.4.6 Acute mitral regurgitation

Typically this occurs 3–5 days post MI, and is generally secondary to rupture of an ischaemic papillary muscle. Acute MR may present with haemodynamic deterioration and/or pulmonary oedema. 25% of cases occur in anterior MI. A murmur is audible in only 50% of cases. A palpable thrill is rare and should raise suspicion of the alternative diagnosis of VSD. Definitive diagnosis by echocardiography is usually straightforward. Additionally, or alternatively, a large 'V' wave can be seen in the pulmonary capillary wedge pressure trace.

Conservative management is associated with a very high mortality: 75% in the first 24 h and at least 90% overall. Emergency mitral valve surgery is the best treatment but nonetheless carries a mortality of 40–90%.

RECOMMENDATIONS

1. Give acute treatment for any pulmonary oedema (✪✪✪ – see section 2.4.1).
2. Once definitive diagnosis is established discuss immediately with local cardiac surgical centre (✪✪✪).
3. Set up sodium nitroprusside infusion at 0.5–10 μg/kg/min (✪ – or GTN if nitroprusside is unavailable).
4. Insert urinary catheter and document renal function (✪).

2.4.7 Post-MI ventricular septal rupture

A post-MI ventricular septal defect (VSD) may present similarly to acute MR. However, two-thirds of cases are associated with anterior MI, a murmur is present in 90% of cases and this is generally associated with a thrill at the left sternal edge. Diagnosis is made by echocardiography or blood gas sampling in the right heart, showing a 'step-up' in oxygenation in the RV. This distinguishes a VSD from acute MR. Echocardiography can locate the defect anatomically, which gives important prognostic information.

Mortality with medical treatment alone is more than 90%. Surgical mortality is about 50%, provided renal function is preserved. The outlook from surgery is much worse in VSD following inferior infarction and some surgical centres feel that conservative or palliative management is the only option in this case.

RECOMMENDATIONS

1. Give acute treatment for any pulmonary oedema (✪✪✪ – see section 2.4.1).
2. Once definitive diagnosis is established, discuss immediately with local cardiac surgical centre (✪✪✪).
3. Set up sodium nitroprusside infusion at 0.5–10 μg/kg/min (✪ – or GTN if nitroprusside is unavailable).
4. Insert urinary catheter and document renal function (✪).

2.4.8 Left ventricular free wall rupture

This occurs in 1–4% of post-MI patients and is almost always rapidly fatal, frequently presenting as chest pain, haemodynamic collapse and electro-mechanical dissociation. Occasionally a rupture is small and contained by the pericardium, forming a pseudoaneurysm with a narrow neck, potentially visible on echocardiography. Such patients should be referred for consideration for surgery since the pseudoaneurysm remains at risk of rupture (✪).

Post-MI VSD appears to be rare in modern practice, comprising only 0.2% of cases in the GUSTO database[48]. Risk factors identified included advanced age, female gender, anterior site of MI and **no** previous smoking history. Medical mortality at 30 days was 94%, patients selected for surgery had a 30 day mortality of 47%.

REFERENCE

48. Crenshaw BS et al (2000) Risk factors, angiographic patterns, and outcomes in patients with ventricular septal defect complicating acute myocardial infarction *Circulation* 101:27–32 (✓✓)

Risk stratification post MI

3.1 Clinical risk stratification

Patients with no early ventricular arrhythmic episodes, no recurrent ischaemic chest pain, preserved BP and preserved LV function (e.g. echocardiographic ejection fraction >50%) are at low risk of a further coronary event.

Assuming these patients mobilise satisfactorily, aim for discharge at 5 days post MI.

A 28 day mortality post MI mortality of less than 1% was predicted in a large Australian study for patients who met all the following criteria

> age <60 years
> heart rate <100/min
> typical symptoms at presentation
> no prior MI
> not diabetic
> no significant Q wave in admission ECG

One-third of 6746 patients studied met all of these criteria[50]. Patients who meet these criteria should be eligible for early discharge, e.g. at 5 days post MI.

> Patients with
>> recurrent ischaemia
>> re-infarction
>> ventricular arrhythmias
>> hypotension
>> cardiac failure
> are at high risk of recurrent events and should be
> referred to a cardiologist prior to discharge from hospital

Recent reviews are available for risk stratification[51] and the pathophysiology[52] of acute coronary syndromes.

Overall in-hospital mortality figures for non-trial MI patients are surprisingly difficult to come by. Most authorities accept that real-world in-hospital mortality for 'all-comers' is 15–25% in the UK, despite the <10% early mortality achieved in the major thrombolytic trials (see e.g. the MONICA data[53]).

In the patients included on the GUSTO database 90% of the early prognostic information was contained in five freely available measures[54].

1. increasing age
2. low blood pressure
3. high Killip class (see Table 2.2)
4. elevated heart rate
5. anterior MI on presenting ECG

A detailed and well validated model based on the GUSTO data is available for predicting 30 day mortality from MI[55]. In practice, this requires a spreadsheet program to calculate an individual's risk, but this is relatively straightforward to set up. This model has not been validated on other patient populations.

REFERENCES

50. Parsons RW et al (1994) Early identification of patients at low risk of death after myocardial infarction and potentially suitable for early hospital discharge *BMJ* 308:1006–1010 (✓✓✓)

51. Timmis A (2000) Coronary disease: Acute coronary syndromes: risk stratification *Heart* 83:241–246 (✓✓✓)

52. Davies MJ (2000) The pathophysiology of acute coronary syndromes *Heart* 83:361–366 (✓✓✓)

53. Tunstall-Pedoe H et al (1996) Sex differences in myocardial infarction and coronary deaths in the Scottish MONICA population of Glasgow 1985 to 1991: Presentation, diagnosis, treatment, and 28-day case fatality of 3991 events in men and 1551 events in women *Circulation* 93:1981–1992 (✓✓)

54. Newby LK et al (1996) Early discharge in the thrombolytic era: an analysis of criteria for uncomplicated infarction from the Global Utilization of streptokinase and t-PA for Occluded Coronary Arteries (GUSTO) trial *JACC* 27:625–632

55. Lee KL et al (1995) Predictors of 30-Day mortality in the era of reperfusion for acute myocardial infarction: Results from an international trial of 41,021 Patients *Circulation* 91:1659–1668 (✓✓✓)

3.2 Using exercise and other 'stress' testing

Patients who are physically capable of performing a treadmill test, and who have ECGs which permit interpretation for ischaemic change during exercise, should have a treadmill exercise test before first out-patient review at 4–6 weeks following discharge (✪✪✪).

The optimal timing of exercise testing in the 'thrombolytic era' has not been determined. Two commonly used approaches are

1. submaximal test at 5–10 days post MI
2. symptom limited test at 14–21 days post MI

Testing at this early stage appears safe if patients have mobilised successfully within hospital, have no symptoms of heart failure or angina and have a stable ECG 48–72 h prior to testing (ACC/AHA).

Local facilities and protocols may decide whether exercise testing is carried out pre-discharge or in the early post-discharge period.

Standard treadmill testing is precluded by LBBB, or persistently abnormal ST-T segment changes on the resting ECG. Such patients should be referred to a Nuclear Medicine department for myocardial perfusion imaging, or for stress echocardiographic studies. In patients unable to exercise pharmacological agents such as adenosine or dobutamine can be used as surrogates.

Patients who are unable to exercise constitute a high risk group of post-MI patients (GISSI-2[56] and TIMI II[57]).

Conversely, patients with negative tests post-thrombolysis have a good prognosis[58]. In 105 post-MI patients with negative exercise tests 97% were free of major events at 6 months follow-up. A Swedish study in 75 patients who were able to exercise 5–8 days post MI concluded that a negative symptom limited test had a better negative predictive value (11% 1 year event rate) than a negative submaximal test (25% 1 year event rate)[59]. A 'submaximal' test is generally stopped if one or more of the following end-points are reached

> Peak heart rate achieved of 70% of predicted maximum for age
> (Usually taken as 220 minus age in years)
> Peak work level of 5 METS
> Development of angina or significant shortness of breath
> ST segment depression >2 mm
> Fall in BP with exercise
> Development of LBBB
> 3 or more consecutive ventricular ectopics
> Development of VT

1 MET (metabolic equivalent) is the energy level required for sitting at rest. 5–7 METS is the energy level required for walking on the flat at 4.5–5 mph, for swimming and for gardening. >9 METS are required for carrying heavy loads up stairs, playing squash or jogging at >6 mph. If the patient has a strenuous job or leisure activity ACC/AHA recommendations are for a second, symptom-limited exercise test at 3–6 weeks post MI (✪✪✪).

REFERENCES

56. Villella A et al (1995) Prognostic significance of maximal exercise testing after myocardial infarction treated with thrombolytic agents: the GISSI-2 database *Lancet* 346:523–529(✓✓✓)

57. Chaitman BR et al (1993) Impact of treatment strategy on predischarge exercise test in the Thrombolysis in Myocardial Infarction (TIMI) II Trial *Am J Cardiol* 71:131–138 (✓✓)

58. Piccalo G et al (1992) Value of negative predischarge exercise testing in identifying patients at low risk after acute myocardial infarction treated by systemic thrombolysis *Am J Cardiol* 70:31–33 (✓)

59. Jensen-Urstad K et al (1999) Prognostic value of symptom limited versus low level exercise stress test before discharge in patients with myocardial infarction treated with thrombolytics *Heart* 82:199–203 (✓)

RECOMMENDATIONS

1. All patients with interpretable ECGs capable of performing treadmill testing should do so within 5–21 days post MI (✪✪✪).

2. Patients who cannot exercise or with ECGs which preclude interpretation should have nuclear perfusion studies or echocardiographic studies as an alternative (✪✪✪).

3. Patients with a negative early exercise test who have a strenuous job or leisure interest should perform an additional symptom-limited test at 3–6 weeks (✪✪✪).

4. Patients with positive exercise tests, or with perfusion scans or echocardiograms suggesting reversible ischaemia should be referred to a cardiologist for coronary angiography (✪✪✪).

3.3 Autonomic markers of post MI risk

There is considerable interest at present in the use of markers of autonomic function such as heart-rate variability (HRV) and baroreflex sensitivity (BRS) as tools for predicting mortality after MI. HRV can be measured non-invasively by analysis of ambulatory 24 h ECG recordings. BRS measurement requires invasive testing such as measuring the rate-pressure response to a phenylephrine infusion.

Despite demonstrations of the utility of abnormal values of autonomic markers as predictors of excess post-MI mortality, their measurement cannot yet be recommended for routine clinical use. Currently available methods of improving autonomic function post MI, such as beta-blockade and exercise, should in any case be part of routine post-MI treatment protocols (see e.g. sections 2.3, 4.1.3 and 6.2.1). Demonstration of abnormal autonomic function post MI does not therefore at present appreciably alter standard management.

In ATRAMI[60] 1284 post-MI patients were studied prospectively. Both low HRV and low BRS were predictors of excess cardiac mortality (odds ratios of 3.2 for HRV and 2.8 for BRS). If both were abnormal, the 2 year mortality was 17%; when both were normal, 2 year mortality was 2%. These measures were independent of left ventricular function as predictors, and gave additional predictive value when used in conjunction with measures of left ventricular function.

The value and limitation of ATRAMI and other studies of autonomic function post MI are discussed by Barron and Viskin[61].

REFERENCES

60. ATRAMI investigators (1998) Baroreflex sensitivity and heart-rate variability in prediction of total cardiac mortality after myocardial infarction *Lancet* 351:478–484 (✓✓✓)

61. Barron HV and Viskin S (1998) Autonomic markers and prediction of cardiac death after myocardial infarction *Lancet* 351:461–462 (✓✓)

3.4 Out-patient follow-up

All patients should be offered at least one out-patient appointment following an MI, and these arrangements should ideally be made prior to discharge (✪✪✪). Medical follow-up is generally undertaken at 6–8 weeks after presentation and offers the clinician a chance to

assess the functional recovery of the patient

assess their clinical state

review their progress in rehabilitation (formal or otherwise)

discuss risk factor modification

check they are on appropriate medication

review investigations such as exercise tests

make further specialist referral if required

Traditionally this is also the time when the patient is 'signed off' as fit to go back to work, if this is relevant.

For the patient this may be the only occasion they have to discuss any factual questions or worries they may have with their hospital doctor.

Hospital out-patient review is also important for the patient's general practitioner in that they can be updated about the patient's clinical state, investigation results and likely outlook.

A checklist for the main points which should be covered during the consultation is given in section 4.3.

Lack of follow-up of post-MI patients appears to be a marker of adverse prognosis. Data from the Nottingham MI registry indicate that patients who were not followed up had a mortality of 50% at 4 years post MI compared to 24% in those who were followed, after correction for age, sex and previous infarction. There was no difference in the proportion of cardiovascular deaths between the two groups[62].

REFERENCE

62. Melville M et al Outcome and use of health services four years after admission for acute myocardial infarction: case record follow up study (1999) *BMJ* 319:230–231 (✓)

3.5 Pre-discharge checklist

Prior to discharge from hospital the following issues should be reviewed
  Smoking
  Blood pressure
  Weight/body mass index

The following drugs should be prescribed in all patients without specific contra-indications

  Beta-blocker
  Aspirin

The following drugs should be prescribed in all patients fulfilling relevant criteria

  ACE inhibitor
  Statin
  Insulin
  Warfarin
  Amiodarone

Clear advice should have been given on the following subjects

  Return to daily activities, including sexual intercourse
  Return to driving
  Return to work
  Risk factor modification

The following arrangements should have been made

  Letter to GP, detailing medications
  Referral for cardiac rehabilitation
  Out-patient exercise test and/or nuclear perfusion study or stress echocardiogram
  Repeat lipid estimation if statin started in hospital
  6–8 week follow-up appointment or cardiology referral

> It is useful to give the patient a copy of a pre-discharge
> ECG in case they re-present acutely

Body mass index is defined as weight (kilograms) divided by the square of height (metres).

Early rehabilitation, secondary prevention and out-patient follow-up of MI

4.1 Cardiac rehabilitation and secondary prevention

The World Health Organisation definition of cardiac rehabilitation is

> 'the sum of activities required to ensure the best possible physical, mental and social conditions, so that the cardiac patient may resume as normal a place as possible in the life of the community'.

A detailed review of cardiac rehabilitation is outside the scope of this manual, although in-hospital measures (WHO phase I) will be considered further. Cardiac rehabilitation is reviewed in depth in e.g. reference 63. Cardiac rehabilitation aims to combine graded exercise training tailored to an individual's capacity and circumstances with education about coronary risk factor modification.

Risk factor intervention post MI is of value since patients with proven coronary artery disease have 5–7 times the event rate of patients with similar risk factors but no overt coronary disease[64].

Non-pharmacological interventions proven to reduce the risk of recurrent events include

1. Stopping smoking
2. Dietary modification
3. Regular physical activity and exercise
4. Weight reduction
5. Alcohol consumption

REFERENCES

63. Supplement O (1998) *Eur Heart J* 19 (✓✓✓)
64. Pekkanen J et al (1990) Ten-year mortality from cardiovascular disease in relation to cholesterol level among men with and without preexisting cardiovascular disease *NEJM* 322:1700–1707 (✓✓✓)

4.1.1 Smoking

There is little or no debate that stopping smoking post MI is beneficial and it may be the most effective single intervention in managing patients post MI.

Most of the evidence comes from the 'pre-thrombolytic' era. Mortality in BHAT at 25 months was 19.8% in those continuing to smoke and 9.9% in those who gave up. The risk of MI in men surviving at least 2 years post MI or unstable angina who give up smoking is approximately halved compared to persistent smokers[65]. In the CASS study the improvement in survival after stopping smoking was comparable to that seen with coronary by-pass surgery[66].

Nicotine patches appear to be a safe and effective adjunct to help smokers quit cigarettes[67].

4.1.2 Diet

Dietary modifications should provide the first approach to lowering raised plasma cholesterol levels, despite the proven prognostic advantage of using HMG-CoA reductase inhibitors to lower plasma cholesterol levels in some post-MI patients.

However, there is increasing evidence that altering dietary intake of oily fish and/or fish oil may reduce mortality independent of any action on total plasma cholesterol levels. For instance, in the DART study of 2033 male post-MI patients, the group taking daily fatty fish had a 29% reduction in all-cause mortality at 2 years, although the incidence of reinfarction plus death from coronary disease at 2 years was not altered[68]. In a smaller French study, a diet reducing levels of red meat, butter and cream and increasing proportions of fruit, green vegetables, bread and canola-based margarine – the so-called Mediterranean diet – also achieved significant reductions in cardiovascular deaths and recurrent MIs[69].

A common theme to these two diets may be increased consumption of omega-3 fatty acids. This is found in high concentrations in oily fish and is produced from linolenic acid which is plentiful in the 'Mediterranean' diet.

The National Service Framework for Coronary Heart Disease in England recommends that dietary advice and statins be used to lower serum cholesterol concentrations EITHER to less than 5 mmol/l (LDL to below 3 mmol/l) OR by 30%, whichever is the greater.

Simvastatin and pravastatin remain the only two HMG-CoA reductase inhibitors proven to offer prognostic benefit in post-MI patients (see section 6.5).

REFERENCES

65. Daly LE et al (1983) Long term effect on mortality of stopping smoking after unstable angina and myocardial infarction *BMJ* 287:324–326 (✓)
66. Hermanson B et al (1988) Beneficial six-year outcome of smoking cessation in older men and women with coronary artery disease. Results from the CASS registry. *NEJM* 319:1365–1369 (✓✓)
67. Fiore MC et al (1994) The effectiveness of the nicotine patch for smoking cessation. A meta-analysis. *JAMA* 271:1940–1947 (✓✓✓)
68. Burr ML et al (1989) Effects of changes in fat, fish, and fibre intakes on death and myocardial reinfarction: diet and reinfarction trial *Lancet* ii 757–761 (✓✓✓)
69. de Lorgeril M et al (1996) Effect of a Mediterranean type of diet on the rate of cardiovascular complications in patients with coronary artery disease. Insights into the cardioprotective effect of certain nutriments *JACC* 28:1103–1108 (✓✓)

4.1.3 Exercise

Two meta-analyses of cardiac rehabilitation programmes involving exercise have supported the proposition that such programmes are beneficial, although exercise itself could not be singled out as a protective factor from these data.

A meta-analysis of 10 randomised trials of cardiac rehabilitation (total n = 4347) showed odds ratios of 0.76 for all-cause mortality (CI 0.63–0.92) and 0.75 for cardiovascular death (CI 0.62–0.93). No difference was shown for recurrent, non-fatal MI[70]. A second study examined 22 trials (total n = 4554) with an average 3 year follow up. The group undergoing rehabilitation had more favourable outcomes when total mortality (odds ratio 0.8, CI 0.66–0.96), cardiovascular mortality (odds ratio 0.78, CI 0.63–0.96) and fatal re-infarction (odds ratio 0.75, CI 0.59–0.95) were considered[71].

Overall, improvement in endurance with regular physical exercise post MI is associated with better survival, reduced risk of sudden death and improved biochemical and psychological parameters[72].

4.1.4 Weight reduction

There is no conclusive proof that obesity is an independent risk factor for coronary artery disease. However, obesity interacts adversely with several other risk factors including hypertension, plasma lipids and diabetic control. Overweight post-MI patients in the Framingham study had an increased long-term risk of re-infarction[73].

Overweight (body mass index >25) patients should therefore be advised to lose weight post MI. Such advice should recommend both dietary and lifestyle changes incorporating the positive benefits of 'protective' diets and increased physical activity described above.

Body mass index is defined as weight (kilograms) divided by the square of height (metres).

REFERENCES

70. Oldridge NB et al (1988) Cardiac rehabilitation after myocardial infarction. Combined experience of randomized clinical trials *JAMA* 260:945–950 (✓✓✓)
71. O'Connor GT et al (1989) An overview of randomized trials of rehabilitation with exercise after myocardial infarction *Circulation* 80:234–244 (✓✓✓)
72. Gohlke H and Gohlke-Bärwolf C (1998) Cardiac rehabilitation: where are we going? *Eur Heart J* 19 (Supplement O):O5–O12 (✓✓)
73. Wong ND et al (1989) Risk factors for long-term coronary prognosis after initial myocardial infarction: the Framingham Study *Am J Epidemiol* 130:469–480 (✓✓)

4.1.5 Alcohol consumption

The protective effect on patients with coronary disease of modest alcohol consumption is well recognised and may be due to alcohol's effect on increasing HDL cholesterol[74], and apolipoprotein AI, and reducing fibrinogen[75]. The type of alcoholic drink seems to be immaterial, but up drinking up to 30 g/day was estimated by Rimm and colleagues to reduce the risk of coronary disease by nearly 25%.

There are fewer data on alcohol's effect post MI. One observational study reported reduced all-cause mortality in men taking two to four alcoholic drinks per week, with possible benefit with intakes from one drink per month to more than two drinks per day[76]. Retrospective analysis from the SOLVD study database (which recruited patients with LV ejection fractions <35%) showed that patients who consumed 1–14 drinks per week showed a modest reduction in all-cause mortality compared to patients taking no alcohol. This apparent protective effect was particularly noticeable on the risk of fatal MI[76a].

RECOMMENDATIONS

1. All patients should stop smoking. Nicotine patches can help patients to do this (✪✪✪).
2. Patients should reduce relative intake of red meat and dairy products and increase intake of oily fish, fresh fruit, green vegetables, bread and margarines high in polyunsaturates (✪✪✪).
3. Patients should be offered a cardiac rehabilitation programme incorporating graded exercise (✪✪).
4. Obese and overweight patients should aim to reduce their BMI below 25 with appropriate dietary modification and exercise (✪✪).
5. Continuation of modest alcohol consumption (e.g. 2–14 drinks per week) can be encouraged (✪✪).

REFERENCES

74. Gaziano JM et al (1999) Type of alcoholic beverage and risk of myocardial infarction *Am J Cardiol* 83:52–57 (✓)

75. Rimm EB et al (1999) Moderate alcohol intake and lower risk of coronary heart disease: meta-analysis of effects on lipids and haemostatic factors *BMJ* 319:1523–1528 (✓✓✓)

76. Muntwyler J et al (1998) Mortality and light to moderate alcohol consumption after myocardial infarction *Lancet* 352:1882–1885 (✓✓✓)

76a. Cooper HA et al (2000) Light-to-moderate alcohol consumption and prognosis in patients with left ventricular systolic dysfunction *JACC* 35:1753–1759 (✓✓)

4.2 Fitness to drive

Many patients are concerned about how ischaemic heart disease will affect their ability to drive. A considerable number will depend on driving to continue their usual employment, and some patients will be vocational drivers. Patients should be informed that it is their own responsiblity to inform DVLA and their insurer of any material change in their health which may affect their capacity to drive. However, satisfactory recovery from uncomplicated MI does not have to be notified (see below).

Detailed advice on whether specific medical conditions restrict or prohibit an individual from driving in the UK is published in:

At a glance guide to the current medical standards of fitness to drive

issued regularly by Drivers Medical Unit, DVLA, Swansea. A version of this document is available on the Internet at www.dvla.gov.uk.

Telephone number for advice is 01792 783686

These medical standards distinguish between

Group 1 drivers
(car, motorcycle and light goods vehicle drivers)

Group 2 drivers
(includes large lorries and buses)

The Medical Commission on Accident Prevention recommends that Group 2 standards are also applied to taxi drivers, and emergency police, fire service and ambulance drivers.

Specific conditions

1. Following myocardial infarction

Group 1

Driving must stop for 4 weeks. Patient may start driving again if there is no other disqualifying condition. DVLA need not be notified unless other reasons exist to do so.

Group 2

Driving to stop for at least 6 weeks. Relicensing may be allowed when symptom free, no other disqualifying conditions exist and first 3 stages of Bruce protocol exercise test can be safely completed, while off cardio-active medication. There must be no symptoms or signs of cardiac dysfunction during the test. Coronary angiography is not specifically required.

2. Angina pectoris – stable or unstable

Group 1

Driving must stop if angina is experienced at rest or at the wheel. Driving is permitted if satisfactory control of symptoms is achieved. DVLA need not be notified.

Group 2

Refusal or revocation of license will be recommended with continuing anginal symptoms. If the patient is free of angina for at least 6 weeks then relicensing may be allowed if the exercise test conditions can be met (see 'Following myocardial infarction' above), and there are no other disqualifying conditions.

3. Following coronary by-pass surgery or coronary angioplasty

See advice for myocardial infarction.

4. Following implant of permanent pacemaker

Group 1

Driving must stop for at least 1 week but may commence after this if no other disqualifying conditions exist.

Group 2

Implant disqualifies patient from driving for 6 weeks. Relicensing may be allowed after this if no other disqualifying conditions exist.

Other cardio-vascular conditions are covered in detail in

At a glance guide to the current medical standards of fitness to drive

4.3 Checklist for out-patient review post MI

History

Site of infarct
Was reperfusion therapy given, and at what interval after symptoms?
In-hospital complications
Angina/SOB post discharge
Functional capacity/progress in rehabilitation classes
Risk factor modification
Co-morbidity e.g. diabetes mellitus

Examination

Heart rate/rhythm
Blood pressure
Evidence of LV dysfunction
Weight/body mass index

Medications

Aspirin
Beta-blocker
ACE inhibitor
Statin
Others where relevant e.g. insulin, amiodarone

Investigations

Lipid profile
Exercise test/nuclear perfusion scan or stress echocardiogram

Future management

Return to work
Further review or specialist referral required?

Check the patient has copy of a recent ECG in case they
re-present acutely

Body mass index is defined as weight (kilograms) divided by the square of height (metres).

Management of other acute coronary syndromes

5.1 Unstable angina

5.1.1 Introduction

Unstable angina pectoris (UAP) can be defined as symptoms of myocardial ischaemia at rest or on minimal exertion without evidence of irreversible myocardial damage.

Different presentations of UAP have been classified with differences in short-term outcome and most frequent treatment modality[76].

Incidence is estimated at 1.0–2.4 cases/1000 population/year so a district general hospital (DGH) with a catchment area of 250 000 could expect 250–600 cases/year.

Clinically it is not possible to distinguish between UAP and non-Q wave MI, and quite often the differentiation may only be made in retrospect.

> The prognosis of UAP is an approximate 10% incidence of
> MI or death at 6 months, half of which will occur acutely.
> It is therefore important to recognise that UAP is not a
> benign condition

A typical DGH might therefore expect to see 12–30 cases progressing acutely to MI or death per year.

5.1.2 Adverse prognostic indicators

1. Prolonged e.g. >20 min rest pain[77]
2. Clinical evidence of LV dysfunction such as S3 or pulmonary oedema
3. Hypotension
4. New mitral regurgitation
5. ST depression >1 mm with pain
6. 'Pseudo'-normalisation of T waves with pain
7. Deep 'arrow-head' T wave inversion in multiple leads

5.1.3 Serum markers

Measurement of serum levels of C reactive protein (CRP) and cardiac troponins, such as troponin T (TnT), at presentation aids with early and late risk stratification. CRP assay is offered by most laboratories although troponin assays are less widely available.

For a review of UAP and other acute coronary syndromes see reference 78.

Definitions and concepts of UAP vary considerably. As with AMI, plaque rupture may be the precipitating event, but the pathophysiology of UAP appears distinct. White (platelet rich) non-occlusive thrombus predominates rather than the occlusive red (red cell and fibrin rich) thrombus seen in AMI. This may be a major reason why fibrinolytic therapy is of little value in UAP.

The pathophysiology of UAP is less well understood than with AMI and the evidence base for treatment strategies is therefore less. However, there is considerable current interest in the field with active controversy about optimal treatment regimens.

'Pseudo-normalisation' refers to inverted T waves becoming upright and thus acquiring an apparently normal appearance. It is the progression from inverted to upright that confirms the abnormality. The significance of pseudo-normalisation is equivalent to that of new inverted T waves.

CRP <1.55 mg/dl is associated with low 14 day mortality (0.3%) and CRP >1.55 mg/dl is predictive of death rates >5% at 14 days[79].

Concomitant measure of TnT ('early positive' versus 'negative' on rapid assay) was shown to refine the risk stratification still further. In a UK study 34% of patients were TnT positive and had significantly elevated rates of coronary end-points for up to 2 years after presentation, including death or revascularisation rates of 53%[80].

REFERENCES

76. Braunwald E (1989) Unstable angina: a classification *Circulation* 80:410–414 *and* (1999) Management of unstable angina based on considerations of aetiology Heart 82 (Supplement I) 15–17 (✓✓)
77. Califf RM et al (1988) Importance of clinical measures of ischemia in the prognosis of patients with documented coronary artery disease *JACC* 11:20–26 (✓✓✓)
78. Theroux P and Fuster V (1998) Acute coronary syndromes: unstable angina and non-Q wave myocardial infarction *Circulation* 97:1195–1206 (✓✓✓)
79. Morrow DA et al (1998) C-reactive protein is a potent predictor of mortality independently of and in combination with troponin T in acute coronary syndromes: a TIMI 11A substudy *JACC* 31:1460–5 (✓✓✓)
80. Stubbs P et al (1996) Prospective study of the role of cardiac troponin T in patients admitted with unstable angina *BMJ* 313:262–264 (✓✓)

5.1.4 Treatment

The aims of treatment are
1. To control symptoms
2. Avoid major complications, e.g. MI or death
3. Prevent future acute coronary events

Medical treatment modalities include
1. Anti-ischaemic
2. Anti-coagulation
3. Anti-platelet
4. Symptom relief

Revascularisation represents more definitive therapy but its timing and which patients should be selected for this treatment remains an area of active research.

5.1.4.1 Anti-ischaemic

Beta-blockade and nitrates are the current mainstay of treatment (✪✪✪). With beta-blocker therapy aim for resting heart rate of 55–70 bpm, usually achievable with e.g. atenolol 25–100 mg OD or metoprolol 25–75 mg BD. If beta-blockers are contra-indicated use verapamil or diltiazem to achieve similar effect (✪). Nicorandil may be effective at relieving ischaemic symptoms if beta-blockade alone is insufficient (✪).

Nitrates should be titrated to relieve pain (✪✪✪). Buccal nitrates have high bio-availability but most units prefer IV nitrates despite the cost and requirement for infusion because of 100% bioavailability and ease of titration.

5.1.4.2 Anti-coagulation

Anti-coagulation will be required for at least 2–5 days (✪✪). With unfractionated IV heparin aim for APTT of 2.0–3.0. This may be surprisingly difficult to achieve within the first 48 h of treatment and requires rigorous monitoring and dose adjustment. Use a locally approved nomogram to determine initial dose, and changes in infusion rate in response to APTT results.

Low molecular weight heparins (LMWH) such as enoxaparin and dalteparin are becoming increasingly used instead of unfractionated heparin (✪✪).

The manufacturer's dosing recommendations are:
Enoxaparin – 1 mg/kg SC 12 hourly for minimum of 2 days.
Dalteparin – 120 IU/kg SC 12 hourly with a maximum of 20,000 IU/day for minimum of 5 days.

Nifedipine has been shown to be delterious when used alone as an anti-ischaemic agent in UAP but appears to be a useful adjunctive agent when used with a beta-blocker.

In the CESAR 2 trial nicorandil was shown to be a safe anti-ischaemic agent with the capacity to reduce episodes of ischaemia and transient arrhythmias[81]. It had no effect on the incidence of MI or death.

LMWHs may be at least as effective as unfractionated heparin, and enoxaparin may be superior (FRISC II, FRISC, FRIC – dalteparin, ESSENCE, TIMI 11B – enoxaparin studies). Meta-analysis has questioned this superiority in patients treated with aspirin and offers no support for using LMWHs for longer than 7 days[81a]. Basic drug cost is considerably more than unfractionated heparin. Overall cost-effectiveness is a matter of considerable debate but published cost-effectiveness analyses have consistently favoured LMWHs[82,83].

Undisputed advantages of LMWHs include more convenient administration (usually SC once daily), more reliable anti-coagulation, and no requirement for APTT monitoring.

REFERENCES

81. Patel DJ et al (1999) Cardioprotection by opening of the K(ATP) channel in unstable angina. Is this a clinical manifestation of myocardial preconditioning? Results of a randomized study with nicorandil. CESAR 2 investigation. Clinical European studies in angina and revascularization *Eur Heart J* 20:51–57 (✓)

81a. Eikelboom JW et al (2000) Unfractionated heparin and low-molecular-weight heparin in acute coronary syndrome without ST elevation: a meta-analysis *Lancet* 355:1936–1942 (✓✓✓)

82. Fox KAA and Bosanquet N (1998) Assessing the UK cost implications of the use of low molecular weight heparin in unstable coronary artery disease *Brit J Cardiol* 5:92–105 (✓✓)

83. Mark DB et al (1998) Economic assessment of low-molecular-weight heparin (enoxaparin) versus unfractionated heparin in acute coronary syndrome patients: results from the ESSENCE randomized trial *Circulation* 97:1702–1707 (✓✓)

5.1.4.3 Anti-platelet

All patients should be treated with aspirin unless a major contra-indication exists (✪✪✪). 75 mg OD is probably adequate. Clopidogrel 75 mg OD is an alternative for the rare patient with a true aspirin allergy.

Abciximab and other glycoprotein IIb/IIIa receptor blockers are new anti-platelet agents, with demonstrable benefits in high-risk patients undergoing revascularisation (see section 6.1.2). They are all very expensive, and cannot yet be recommended for routine treatment of UAP in the DGH. If the patient is at high risk of progressing to infarction, or is planned for transfer for PTCA or CABG, discuss their use with the local cardiac centre.

5.1.4.4 Symptom relief

Oxygenation should be optimised e.g. keep oximetry SaO_2 >96% (✪✪✪).

Chest pain should be promptly relieved (✪✪✪). If pain is not relieved within 5–10 min by increasing nitrates, give diamorphine 2.5–10 mg IV incrementally with an anti-emetic. An ECG should be performed with any episode of recurrent ischaemic pain.

Anxiety is often under-estimated as a provocatory factor of chest pain. Reassurance and high-quality nursing are probably the best interventions. Some patients will require anxiolytics e.g. diazepam 1–2 mg PO TDS (✪).

Disrupted sleep is common in the CCU. Earplugs or the patient's usual nightcap may be at least as effective as night sedation with benzodiazepines (✪).

The use of platelet glycoprotein IIb/IIIa inhibitors in acute coronary syndromes with or without subsequent PTCA is an area of considerable current research. Despite several authors' enthusiasm, (see e.g. reference 84) no clinically available agent has been shown to produce benefit beyond 30 days in a prospective, randomised trial unless the patient proceeds to PTCA. Sustained benefit has been shown where the unstable patient has undergone PTCA following use of these agents. Abciximab, tirofiban and eptifibatide are the only agents of this type currently available in the UK. They are all very expensive, and while their cost-effectiveness remains to be demonstrated, it may be favourable and this is an area of much current interest[85].

Pain causes tachycardia, raises blood pressure, increases myocardial workload and oxygen consumption and increases catecholamine release and sympathetic activation. All these effects are detrimental in UAP and may predispose to progression to infarction or to arrhythmias.

REFERENCES

84. Ronner E et al (1998) Platlet glycoprotein IIb/IIIa receptor antagonists. An asset for treatment of unstable coronary syndromes and coronary intervention *Eur Heart J* 19:1608–1616 (✓✓✓)

85. Szucs TD et al (1999) Economic assessment of tirofiban in the management of acute coronary syndromes in the hospital setting: an analysis based on the PRISM PLUS trial *Eur Heart J* 20:1253–1260 (✓✓); Mark DB et al (2000) Cost-effectiveness of platelet glycoprotein IIb/IIIa inhibition with eptifibatide in patients with non-ST-elevation acute coronary syndromes *Circulation* 2000 101:366–371 (✓✓✓); Topol EJ et al for the EPISTENT investigators (1999) Outcomes at 1 year and economic implications of platelet glycoprotein IIb/IIIa blockade in patients undergoing coronary stenting: results from a multicentre randomised trial. EPISTENT Investigators. Evaluation of Platelet IIb/IIIa Inhibitor for Stenting *Lancet* 354: 2019–2124 (✓✓)

5.1.5 Coronary angiography and revascularisation

Definitive therapy for the high-risk patient or for medically refractory symptoms will require PTCA or CABG. Both these approaches require prior coronary angiography to determine coronary anatomy. It remains a challenge to predict which patients will settle and which will require acute intervention.

The risks of acute intervention in patients with acute coronary syndromes are almost certainly higher than in patients who have stablised. So-called 'aggressive' strategies of performing coronary angiography in the majority of patients with acute coronary syndromes have not always been shown to be superior to more conservative 'ischaemia-directed' management[86].

More recent evidence has supported a strategy of early invasive angiography and revascularisation has advantages over a more conservative strategy of early medical treatment, halving the incidence of anginal symptoms and re-admission[87] (✪✪).

> Individual cases should therefore continue to be discussed
> on their merits with the local cardiac centre

On current evidence, the role of the cardiac catheter laboratory in these syndromes has therefore been described as 'unsettled'[88], not least because such technologies as coronary stents and platelet glycoprotein IIb/IIIa inhibitors are emerging faster than trials can evaluate their worth.

REFERENCES

86. Yusuf S et al (1998) Variations between countries in invasive cardiac procedures and outcomes in patients with suspected unstable angina or myocardial infarction without initial ST elevation. OASIS (Organisation to Assess Strategies for Ischaemic Syndromes) Registry Investigators *Lancet* 352:507–514 (✓✓); Boden WE et al (1998) Outcomes in patients with acute non-Q wave myocardial infarction randomly assigned to an invasive as compared with a conservative management strategy. Veterans Affairs Non-Q Wave Infarction Strategies in Hospital (VANQWISH) Trial Investigators *NEJM* 338:1785–1792 (✓✓)

87. Invasive compared with non-invasive treatment in unstable coronary artery disease: FRISC II prospective randomised multicentre study. FRagmin and Fast Revascularisation during InStability in Coronary artery disease Investigators (1999) *Lancet* 354:708–715 (✓✓)

88. Topol E (1998) What role for catheter laboratories in unstable angina? *Lancet* editorial 352:500–501 (✓✓)

5.1.6 Recommendations

On admission to CCU

Bedrest

Medical treatment
1. Anti-ischaemic
2. Anti-coagulation
3. Anti-platelet
4. Symptom relief

Risk-stratify using clinical, ECG, and serum markers. Discuss high-risk patients with senior colleagues and liaise with the local cardiac centre with regard to treatment and/or early transfer.

Each day

Review patient symptoms and haemodynamics
ECGs with pain, and routinely each morning
Measure APTT if on unfractionated heparin. Aim for APTT 2.0–3.0
Measure CK or other serum marker of infarction

If patient not setting

Review history and repeat examination to rule out other causes of symptoms.
Review treatment. Ensure adequately beta-blocked, adequately anti-coagulated and on anti-platelet agent.
Review available investigations, particularly ECGs and serum markers of MI.
If clinical diagnosis is secure and angina remains refractory to treatment refer to local cardiac centre. Local protocols may suggest treatment with glycoprotein IIb/IIIa inhibitors at this stage.

If patient appearing to settle

Continue anti-coagulation for minimum of 48 h total.
Wean off IV nitrates over next 12–24 h.
If symptom-free off IV nitrates begin to mobilise using a post-MI protocol or similar. Continue oral anti-anginal agents.
If symptom-free for 24 h off IV nitrates stop heparin. Continue mobilisation.

Optimal strategies for managing UAP have not been determined and are an area of considerable current interest. The recommendations suggested opposite are based on the available evidence, as outlined above, and the author's current practice.

For a review of risk stratification in acute coronary syndromes see reference 89.

REFERENCE

89. Timmis A (2000) Acute coronary syndromes: risk stratification *Heart* 83:241–246 (✓✓✓)

If symptoms recur during mobilisation

Put back on bedrest, heparin and IV nitrates.
Wean nitrates after further 24–36 h and attempt mobilisation again. If symptoms recur once more, refer to local cardiac centre as medically refractory.

If mobilisation successful

Perform pre-discharge exercise test using local post MI protocol e.g. modified Bruce.
Refer patients with tests positive in stage 1 or 2 for consideration of in-patient coronary angiography. Tests positive later in the protocol can be referred to cardiologist for out-patient review.
Refine risk stratification with pre-discharge CRP level.

5.1.7 MI following unstable angina

The natural history of unstable angina is either to settle or progress to MI. Patients found to have progressed to MI should be treated as such (see section 1). Further unstable symptoms after established myocardial damage mandates referral for consideration of early coronary angiography (✪✪).

5.1.8 Post-discharge management

Overall strategy is similar to the post MI patient.
All eligible patients should be on aspirin and a beta-blocker and have access to sublingual nitrates for use as required. Further oral anti-anginal agents may be required to control anginal symptoms.

Reduction of risk factors to prevent or slow disease progression is important and almost certainly underemphasised. Use of a pre-discharge check-list (see section 5.3) will help systematic review of the major issues which should be addressed after discharge.

A small series of 53 patients has suggested that recurrent clinically significant episodes of ischaemia can be predicted by discharge levels of CRP, with 69% of those with levels >8.7 mg/l requiring re-admission within 3 months[90].

REFERENCE

90. Biasucci LM et al (1999) Elevated levels of C-reactive protein at discharge in patients with unstable angina predict recurrent instability *Circulation* 99:855–860 (✓)

5.2 Non-Q wave MI

5.2.1 Introduction

Although non-Q wave MI is pathologically similar to a Q wave MI the clinical presentation and immediate treatment forms a spectrum with UAP. It is useful to regard non-Q wave MI as an unstable syndrome, rather than as a completed 'small' infarct.

Compared to patients with Q wave MI, patients with non-Q wave MI have

> smaller infarcts
> a better acute prognosis
> similar or worse long-term prognosis
> 2 × risk of recurrent angina
> (Thompson)

Prompt treatment of an acute MI with reperfusion therapy may limit myocardial damage sufficiently to prevent a Q wave MI and it is important that any gain in short-term prognosis should not be squandered by inadequate follow-up.

RECOMMENDATIONS

1. Once non-Q wave MI has been diagnosed treat on CCU as for a Q wave MI although note thrombolysis is not indicated (✪).
2. Early risk stratification with exercise testing, nuclear perfusion studies, stress echocardiography or coronary angiography is important. A pre-discharge exercise test is adequate in most cases (✪✪✪).
3. As with Q wave MI, all patients should receive aspirin and beta-blockers unless there is a major contra-indication (✪✪✪).
4. Modifiable risk factors for future coronary events should be treated as for Q wave MI – see also section 4.1 (✪✪✪).

The pathogenesis of non-Q wave MI is similar to Q wave MI. However, it seems in non-Q wave infarctions there is either spontaneous re-canalisation, or the occluded artery subtends myocardium which has a significant collateral supply[91]. The infarction is usually therefore not transmural although it is inaccurate to equate a non-Q wave MI with an anatomically subendocardial infarction[92].

Risk stratification in non-Q wave MI using the ECG at presentation was examined in the TIMI-III Registry[93], showing that ST deviation as little as 0.5 mm was an adverse prognostic indicator, as was LBBB. Isolated T wave inversion had no predictive value.

Retrospective analysis of over 200,000 patients treated for AMI in the USA has shown approximately 40% mortality reduction in patients treated with beta-blockers[94]. This benefit was also seen in patients with non-Q wave infarcts.

REFERENCES

91. Huey BL et al (1987) Acute non-Q wave myocardial infarction associated with early ST segment elevation: evidence for spontaneous coronary reperfusion and implications for thrombolytic trials *JACC* 9:18–25 (✓✓)
92. Andre-Fouet X (1989) 'Non-Q wave,' alias 'nontransmural,' myocardial infarction: a specific entity *Am Heart J* 117:892–902 (✓✓)
93. Cannon CP et al (1997) The electrocardiogram predicts one-year outcome of patients with unstable angina and non-Q wave myocardial infarction: results of the TIMI III Registry ECG Ancillary Study *JACC* (1997) 30: 133–140 (✓✓)
94. Gottlieb SS et al (1998) Effect of beta-blockade on mortality among high-risk and low-risk patients after myocardial infarction *NEJM* 339:489–497 (✓✓✓)

5.3 Pre-discharge checklist

The following risk factors should be reviewed
> Smoking
> Serum lipids
> Blood pressure
> Weight/body mass index

The following drugs should be prescribed in all patients without specific contra-indications

> Beta-blocker
> Aspirin
> Statin if total cholesterol >5.2 mmol/l
> Sub-lingual nitrates (for PRN and prophylactic use)

Clear advice should have been given on the following subjects

> Return to daily activities, including sexual intercourse
> Return to work, if relevant
> Risk factor modification
> Prophylactic use of nitrates
> When to seek medical attention if symptoms change

The following arrangements should have been made

> Letter to GP, detailing medications
> Exercise test, nuclear perfusion study or stress echocardiogram, if not performed as in-patient
> Repeat lipid estimation if statin started in hospital
> Follow-up appointment or cardiology referral

> **It is useful to give the patient a copy of a pre-discharge ECG in case they re-present acutely**

Body mass index is defined as weight (kilograms) divided by the square of height (metres).

Drugs in common use in MI and unstable angina

6.1 Aspirin and other anti-platelet agents

6.1.1 Aspirin

Aspirin irreversibly inhibits the action of cyclo-oxygenase in platelets, thereby inhibiting platelet thromboxane A_2 synthesis and platelet aggregation. Restoration of platelet function depends on new platelet synthesis by bone marrow. A single dose of aspirin can therefore inhibit platelet function for an entire platelet lifespan of 7–10 days.

Soluble aspirin at a dose of at least 150 mg achieves near total inhibition of platelet thromboxane A_2. Initial dose in acute settings should therefore be at least 150 mg. Maintenance doses higher than 75 mg OD are associated with increased gastro-intestinal side-effects. For chronic use 75 mg appears sufficient to achieve complete cyclo-oxygenase inhibition.

Cardiac settings in which aspirin is of proven benefit [95]

Acute MI

Trial overviews have estimated aspirin prevents 38 major vascular events (i.e. a combined end-point of non-fatal MI, stroke or death) per 1000 patients treated. ISIS-2 showed this effect was independent of the effect of streptokinase and equivalent to the benefit of streptokinase treatment.

Secondary prevention post MI

Absolute benefit is similar to that of treatment in the acute setting with overviews suggesting 36 major vascular events prevented per 1000 patients treated for 2 years (Thompson).

Unstable angina and non-Q wave MI

In other acute coronary syndromes aspirin prevents about 49 major vascular events per 1000 patients treated.

For a detailed analysis of the relative and absolute benefits for various vascular outcomes with aspirin therapy see reference 95.

REFERENCE

95. Antiplatelet Trialists' Collaboration (1994) Collaborative overview of randomised trials of antiplatelet therapy. Prevention of death, myocardial infarction, and stroke by prolonged antiplatelet therapy in various categories of patients *BMJ* 308:81–106 (✓✓✓)

Post CABG and PTCA

Early vascular graft or coronary artery occlusion post PTCA is significantly reduced by aspirin with 93 events prevented per 1000 patients treated for 6 months.

Atrial fibrillation not related to valve disease

The SPAF and SPAF II trials showed that 325 mg aspirin/day reduced the risk of ischaemic stroke in non-rheumatic AF, especially in the under 75 age group, although not by as much as did warfarin. A similar result was found in the EAFT trial in patients with AF who had already suffered a transient ischaemic attack or minor stroke. 300 mg aspirin/day prevented 40 vascular events per year per 1000 patients treated. Warfarin prevented 90 vascular events per year per 1000 patients treated. Aspirin may therefore be an alternative to anti-coagulation in some patients who are not candidates for warfarin.

6.1.2 Glycoprotein IIb/IIIa inhibitors

The prototypical agent in this novel group of anti-platelet agents is abciximab. Glycoprotein IIb/IIIa inhibitors act by blocking the glycoprotein IIb and IIIa receptors on the platelet surface, reducing the ability of platelets to aggregate and form thrombus. Although tirofiban and eptifibatide are now both available in the UK, there is considerably more routine clinical experience with abciximab.

Biochemically, abciximab comprises the Fab (antigen-binding) fragment of a monoclonal antibody to the IIb/IIIa receptor. Since it lacks the Fc antibody fragment it is virtually non-immunogenic. In common with most drugs manufactured via recombinant gene technology it is extremely expensive.

Existing evidence supports the use of abciximab in high-risk PTCA or coronary stenting procedures as a 'one-off' adjunctive treatment. There is accumulating evidence (e.g. EPISTENT) to support its use in all coronary interventional procedures, although no unit in the UK, and possibly none in Europe, can currently justify this approach on grounds of cost. Several trials are under way examining the value of abciximab and other IIb/IIIa blockers in acute coronary syndromes. Current practice in the UK therefore virtually limits its use to interventional centres, although some centres are piloting the use of glycoprotein IIb/IIIa inhibitors for acute coronary syndromes in district centres prior to transfer for PTCA. Such use is likely to increase in the future.

The development, pharmacology and clinical use of platelet glycoprotein IIb/IIIa inhibitors are discussed in detail in references 96 and 97.

REFERENCES

96. Topol EJ et al (1999) Platelet GPIIb-IIIa blockers *Lancet* 353:227–231 (✓✓✓)
97. Ronner E et al (1998) Platelet glycoprotein IIB/IIIA receptor antagonists. An asset for treatment of unstable coronary syndromes and coronary intervention *Eur Heart J* 19:1608–1616 (✓✓✓)

Abciximab has also been used as adjunctive anti-platelet therapy with aspirin, tPA and heparin in a reperfusion regimen used to treat acute MI in the TIMI-14 trial[98]. This type of reperfusion therapy may well continue to gain acceptance if further evidence accumulates to support its use.

Abciximab is given as a bolus, followed by a 12 h infusion. The dose is weight dependent. Since IIb/IIIa GP inhibitors are used relatively infrequently the manufacturer's dosing recommendations should be consulted at each use.

Concomitant heparin therapy should be adjusted to give an activated clotting time of under 200 s. The major drawback to the use of abciximab is of excessive bleeding complications, often from femoral artery puncture sites post-intervention, with concomitant heparin therapy. The reported frequency of severe thrombocytopaenia (platelet count below 50/nl) is 0.5–1.6%. There appears to be no excess of intracranial haemorrhage with abciximab treatment.

RECOMMENDATIONS

1. Abciximab and other platelet glycoprotein IIb/IIIa inhibitors cannot yet be recommended for routine use in treating acute coronary syndromes in district hospitals (✪✪).
2. The use of glycoprotein IIb/IIIa inhibitors may be justified in unstable coronary syndromes where early transfer to an interventional centre can be guaranteed (✪✪).
3. At present there is no evidence to suggest tirofiban or eptifibatide are superior to abciximab in acute coronary syndromes (✪✪).

REFERENCE

98. Antman EM et al (1999) Abciximab facilitates the rate and extent of thrombolysis: results of the Thrombolysis In Myocardial Infarction (TIMI) 14 Trial *Circulation* 99:2720–2732 (✓✓)

6.2 Beta-blockers

6.2.1 Benefits of beta-blockade in acute MI

There is little doubt that long term use of beta-blockers improves survival in patients who have had myocardial infarction, the main evidence coming from 1980s trials.

A systematic review of randomised controlled trials, comprising a total of over 54,000 patients, identified an odds ratio of death from long-term trials of 0.77 (CI 0.69–0.85), with an estimated annual reduction of 12 deaths/1000 patients treated/year[99]. This review found that the agents with most evidence to support their use were propranolol, metoprolol and timolol.

Retrospective analysis of over 200,000 patients treated for AMI in the USA has shown approximately 40% mortality reduction in patients treated with beta-blockers[100]. Unexpectedly and importantly this benefit was also seen in patients with non-Q wave infarcts and with obstructive airways disease, both having traditionally been regarded as definite contra-indications to beta-blocker use. Smaller relative, but similar absolute, benefits were found in other groups in whom beta-blocker usage is traditionally low e.g. patients >80 years old, LVEF <20%, and patients with renal impairment or with diabetes. Beta-blockers are almost certainly under-used so that many patients who would benefit from them do not receive them (ASPIRE, EUROASPIRE, Gottlieb et al above).

Controversial issues include

1. the optimal timing of starting beta-blocker therapy
2. the route of initial administration
3. what constitutes a contra-indication to their use

Class I recommendations (ACC/AHA) for use of beta-blockers in the setting of AMI exists for

1. Patients without a contra-indication to beta-blocker therapy who can be treated within 12 h of onset of infarction, irrespective of reperfusion therapy with thrombolytics or primary angioplasty (✪✪✪).
2. Patients with continuing or recurrent ischaemic pain (✪✪✪).
3. Patients with tachycardias, such as AF with a rapid ventricular response (✪✪✪)
4. Non-ST-elevation MI (✪✪✪).

REFERENCES

99. Freemantle N et al (1999) Beta blockade after myocardial infarction: systematic review and meta regression analysis *BMJ* 318: 1730–1737 (✓✓✓)
100. Gottlieb SS et al (1998) Effect of beta-blockade on mortality among high-risk and low-risk patients after myocardial infarction *NEJM* 339:489–497 (✓✓✓)

Early beta-blocker therapy appears to

1. Reduce rate of reinfarction when thrombolytics are used
2. Reduce infarct size and complications when thrombolytics are not used (ACC/AHA)

6.2.2 Intravenous beta-blockade in MI

This method of administration has generally fallen out of favour in the UK. IV beta-blockers were used in e.g. the ISIS-1, MIAMI and TIMI-II trials. Benefits were relatively small (~6 lives saved per 1000 patients treated in pre-thrombolytic trials). It is reasonable, but of uncertain benefit, to use IV agents in patients presenting with tachycardia, hypertension or pain unresponsive to opioids (✪✪ – Euro).

Dose regimens of proven value include

Atenolol 5–10 mg IV, followed by 100 mg/day PO
(✪✪✪ – ISIS-1)
Metoprolol 15 mg IV, followed by 50 mg BD, PO, increasing to 100 mg BD (✪✪✪ – TIMI-II)

Some authorities argue for early intravenous treatment with beta-blockers in MI, followed by chronic oral therapy. The issue is complicated by the advent of thrombolytic therapy since much of the evidence supporting early intravenous use comes from the 'pre-thrombolytic' era.

The validity of more generally applying the available trial evidence of the benefits of IV beta-blockers has also been called into question. In most trials, only small proportions of patients received IV beta-blockers in the UK, especially when compared to other countries. Figures in the UK ranged from 0.2% to 5% with figures of 30–54% in countries such as Italy, Sweden and the USA. It may not therefore be reasonable to generalise any results to the wider MI population in the UK.

6.2.3 Initial intravenous vs initial oral treatment

There is no good evidence that giving intravenous beta-blockers early is superior to giving oral beta-blockers early. However, most of the evidence showing benefit from early beta-blockade comes from trials which included initial IV administration. That caution should be exercised with such regimens is suggested by analysis of the GUSTO-I database. This showed definite benefits with beta-blocker treatment but higher mortality amongst those whose regimen included initial IV atenolol[101].

What can be concluded about beta-blocker use in the setting of AMI?
1. They are haemodynamically safe in the very earliest stages of AMI, even when given intravenously.
2. The benefit is significant, typically improving survival by 40% and is spread across many patient groups.
3. At least some patients with 'contra-indications' to beta-blockade appear to benefit from their use.
4. They are very cost-effective.

RECOMMENDATIONS

1. Patients with haemodynamic indications of high adrenergic drive e.g. high BP and HR can be treated immediately with either IV or oral beta-blockers, and with thrombolysis if eligible (✪✪✪).
2. Every patient with confirmed Q wave or non-Q wave MI should be given beta-blocker therapy within 12 h of presentation unless a firm contra-indication exists. Many patients can therefore be assessed for beta-blocker therapy the morning following admission (✪✪✪).
3. Where a contra-indication to beta-blockade is thought to exist the relative risk-benefit of treating in any case with beta-blockers should be specifically assessed. For instance it may be reasonable to give a patient with COAD a trial of cardioselective beta-blocker and re-assess lung function and respiratory symptoms shortly after starting therapy (✪✪).
4. Where beta-blockers are withheld the reason for doing so should be clearly documented to assist future decisions about therapy (✪✪✪).

It follows that **every** post-MI patient should either be given beta-blockers or have documented a good reason why not. This situation is similar to that recommended for thrombolytic therapy.

A detailed review of randomised trials of beta-blockade in MI found that initial intravenous therapy gave no additional benefit[102].

Some uncontrolled data exist to suggest lower doses of beta-blocker may be as least as effective as the relatively high doses used in large trials[103].

Viewpoints

'The case for IV beta blockade in patients who do not receive reperfusion treatment is secure, but for those treated with thrombolysis or primary angioplasty the data are far from overwhelming'
Ludman PF (1999) *BMJ* 318:328

'Early IV atenolol seems of limited value. The best approach for most patients may be to begin oral atenolol once stable'
Pfisterer M et al (1998) *JACC* 32:634–640

REFERENCES

101. Pfisterer M et al (1998) Atenolol use and clinical outcomes after thrombolysis for acute myocardial infarction: the GUSTO-I experience. Global Utilization of Streptokinase and TPA (alteplase) for Occluded Coronary Arteries *JACC* 32:634–640 (✓✓✓)

102. Freemantle N et al (1999) Beta blockade after myocardial infarction:-systematic review and meta regression analysis *BMJ* 318:1730–1737 (✓✓✓)

103. Barron HV et al (1998) Beta-blocker dosages and mortality after myocardial infarction: data from a large health maintenance organization *Arch Int Med* 158:449–453 (✓)

6.3 Calcium channel blockers

Calcium channel blockers have only a relatively small part to play following MI or other acute coronary syndromes, with trials showing only modest benefits and considerable problems. Despite their common pharmacological action, individual agents show distinct properties which are almost certainly clinically relevant. Chief amongst these are effects on heart rate, and on left ventricular function.

No trial of a calcium channel blocker post MI has shown a reduction in overall mortality. Trends to reducing mortality are more favourable with agents which limit heart rate such as verapamil (e.g. DAVIT II) or diltiazem (MDPIT) than in those which tend to cause reflex tachycardia. Immediate release nifedipine appears to be detrimental when used without a beta-blocker post MI (e.g. SPRINT). Amlodipine has not been specifically examined post MI but appears to be safe in patients with impaired LV function (PRAISE).

The question of whether to use a calcium channel blocker post MI is often raised where beta-blockers are thought to be contra-indicated and an anti-ischaemic agent or ventricular rate control is required. However, it is clear that beta-blockers are prognostically beneficial even in many patients with factors traditionally regarded as contra-indications[104]. The best option in such patients may therefore be to re-assess the contra-indication and use beta-blockers if at all possible – see section 6.2.4.

If beta-blockers have been ruled out post MI it seems reasonable to limit the choice of calcium channel blocker to a rate-limiting agent, since this may be part of the way beta-blockers confer benefit. Verapamil is probably the best choice in survivors of Q wave MI, particularly if LV function is good. Diltiazem should be avoided if the patient shows evidence of pulmonary oedema.

In non-Q wave MI with no evidence of heart failure, both diltiazem and verapamil have been shown to reduce cardiac mortality (MDPIT and DAVIT II).

Viewpoint

'Calcium channel blockers have not proven beneficial in early treatment or secondary prevention of acute MI, and the possibility of harm has been raised. In patients with first non–Q wave infarction or first inferior infarction without LV dysfunction or pulmonary congestion, verapamil and diltiazem may reduce the incidence of reinfarction, but their benefit beyond that of β-adrenoceptor blockers and aspirin is unclear. Similarly, there are no data to support the use of second-generation dihydropyridines (e.g. amilodipine, felodipine) for improving survival in acute MI'
(ACC/AHA).

In DAVIT II patients with evidence of heart failure post MI treated with verapamil showed no evidence of increased rates of mortality or re-infarction at 18 months. In contrast, in MDPIT patients with chest X-ray evidence of pulmonary oedema had significantly increased rates of death and re-infarction when treated with diltiazem rather than placebo.

REFERENCE

104. Gottlieb SS et al (1998) Effect of beta-blockade on mortality among high-risk and low-risk patients after myocardial infarction *NEJM* 339:489–497 (✓✓✓)

RECOMMENDATIONS

1. Use calcium channel blockers post MI only in conjunction with a beta-blocker (this excludes verapamil), or where a beta-blocker is definitively contra-indicated (✪✪).

2. In Q wave infarction with pulmonary oedema limit the choice to amlodipine or verapamil. Do not use verapamil in patients with heart failure during the first 24–48 h post MI. Use a nitrate instead if possible (✪✪).

3. In Q wave infarction with no pulmonary oedema diltiazem or verapamil may be used (✪✪).

4. In non-Q wave MI with no pulmonary oedema diltiazem or verapamil may be used (✪✪✪).

5. Avoid nifedipine in the post MI patient (✪✪).

6. Calcium channel blockers may generally be used safely in acute coronary syndromes when used with a beta-blocker (✪✪).

ACC/AHA guidelines (✪✪ – **Class IIa recommendation**) also suggest the following uses for verapamil or diltiazem: Control of ongoing ischaemia or ventricular rate control in fast AF where a beta-blocker is contra-indicated and there is no heart failure, LV dysfunction or AV block.

There are no Class I recommendations.

6.4 ACE inhibitors

There is ACC/AHA Class I evidence (❸❸❸) of clinical benefit for post MI use of the following ACE inhibitors available in the UK.

Agent	Major trial evidence	Calculated early lives saved/1000 patients treated
Captopril	ISIS-4	5
Lisinopril	GISSI-3	8
Ramipril	AIRE(X)	21
Trandolapril	TRACE	24

In ISIS-4 and GISSI-3, ACE inhibitors were begun on day 0 in unselected patients. In both AIRE and TRACE, patients were selected on the basis of LV function and treatment was delayed until at least day 3. This may account for the apparent superiority of ramipril and trandolapril since their use was 'focused' on patients with evident LV dysfunction.

Note that enalapril is not included, and in CONSENSUS II was shown not to be of benefit post MI, when given as the pro-drug enalaprilat.

The evidence therefore suggests two possible strategies when using ACE inhibitors post MI (❸❸❸):

i. Early unselective treatment

The first is to give ACE inhibitors to all patients at day 0, reviewing the need for them at 6 week follow-up and continuing them only in those patients with residual evidence of LV dysfunction. The main advantage of this approach is that it offers all patients the early benefits of ACE inhibition. Since ~50% of deaths prevented by ACE inhibitors occur in the first week post MI this is potentially valuable. The major disadvantage of this strategy is its lack of specificity. All patients are exposed not only to the benefits, but also to the risks and side-effects of ACE inhibitors. There are also considerable cost implications and the cost-effectiveness of this strategy has not been examined.

Contra-indications to ACE inhibitor therapy include

1. Hypotension e.g. systolic BP <90 mmHg
2. Bilateral renal artery stenosis
3. Renal impairment, not yet dialysis dependent
4. Angio-oedema or other limiting side-effects with previous ACE inhibitor treatment

Selecting appropriate patients and optimal timing of ACE inhibitor therapy is discussed in reference 105.

REFERENCE

105. Pfeffer MA (1998) ACE inhibitors in acute myocardial infarction: patient selection and timing *Circulation* 97:2192–2194 (✓✓✓)

ii. Later selective treatment

The second strategy is to select those patients with evidence of LV dysfunction in the first days after MI and continue them on ACE inhibitors long term. AIREX suggests this benefit is maintained at least 5 years post MI.

Very recent evidence from the HOPE study has suggested that all patients with coronary artery disease may benefit from long-term treatment with ramipril, and this would include all post-MI patients. The cost-effectiveness of this strategy has yet to be fully evaluated.

RECOMMENDATIONS

1. Patients with anterior Q wave MI, or early overt evidence of LV dysfunction (clinical, radiological or echo ejection fraction <40%) should receive ACE inhibitors within 24 h post MI (✪✪✪).
2. Other patients can be reassessed for evidence of LV dysfunction at 48–72 h post MI, and commenced on an ACE inhibitor at that time (✪✪✪).
3. Patients with non-anterior Q wave MI, normal ejection fraction and no residual evidence of LV dysfunction may have ACE inhibitors stopped at 6 week follow-up (✪).
4. Patients selected for treatment should continue to receive ACE inhibitors for at least 5 years post MI and probably life-long (✪✪✪).

Note that an indication for ACE inhibition does not imply a contra-indication to beta-blockade. In appropriately selected patients, the combined use of ACE inhibitors and beta-blockers is probably beneficial via separate mechanisms.

Suggested regimens (depending on adequate BP)

Captopril	25–50 mg TDS
Lisinopril	10 mg OD
Ramipril	2.5–5 mg BD
Trandolapril	2–4 mg OD

Consensus statements and reviews

'The following groups of patients should be given ACE inhibitors post MI:
1. Patients within the first 24 h of a suspected acute MI with ST-segment elevation in two or more anterior precordial leads or with clinical heart failure in the absence of significant hypotension (systolic blood pressure <100 mmHg) or known contra-indications to use of ACE inhibitors.
2. Patients with MI and LV ejection fraction less than 40% or patients with clinical heart failure on the basis of systolic pump dysfunction during and after convalescence from acute MI.'
ACC/AHA – Class I recommendation

'All patients with AMI with evidence of LV impairment, or other risk factors such as anterior infraction, left bundle branch block or history of previous MI should receive early (within 24 h) treatment with oral ACE inhibitors' Dana and Walker (1999)[106].

REFERENCE

106. Dana A and Walker M (1999) Acute myocardial infarction. Extended review *J Roy Coll Phys Lond* 33:131–140

6.5 Lipid-lowering agents

Blood should be taken for serum lipid estimation on admission with suspected MI. The stress of AMI lowers serum lipid levels below baseline. If an admission sample is not taken at least 4 weeks should elapse before levels of total cholesterol, LDL and HDL cholesterols and triglycerides have recovered sufficiently to make decisions about treatment[107].

Lipid-lowering therapy with either of two HMG CoA reductase inhibitors ('statins') has been shown to reduce mortality in patients with established coronary artery disease. These are simvastatin (e.g. '4S' study) and pravastatin (e.g. CARE), see Table 6.1.

No other statin agents have shown improved outcome with cholesterol lowering in comparable populations. 4S included patients with stable angina, the CARE study population was limited to survivors of MI. These trial data suggest simvastatin treatment for 6 years saves 40 deaths from CAD and 7 non-fatal MIs per 1000 patients treated, and that pravastatin treatment for 5 years saves 11 CAD deaths and 26 non-fatal MIs per 1000 patients treated[108].

Most UK clinicians use lower initial doses of these agents post MI. This is in line with the philosophy of the 4S study which aimed to titrate dose to achieve a total cholesterol between 3.0 and 5.2 mmol/l. Atorvastatin is probably the most cost-effective agent in terms of cholesterol lowering but as yet there are no outcome data to support its use post MI.

RECOMMENDATIONS

1. All patients with MI should have serum lipids measured (✪✪✪).
2. Simvastatin or pravastatin should be given to any post-MI patient with LDL >3.3 or total cholesterol >4.8. Economic considerations may dictate an initial dose of 10 mg/day (✪✪✪).
3. Other factors affecting serum cholesterol (diet, smoking, diabetes etc.) should be simultaneously addressed (✪✪✪).
4. Response to lipid-lowering therapy should be followed up with dose increase to maximum of 40 mg/day of either agent as required. Poor responders, or those with complex hyperlipidaemias, require referral to a lipid clinic (✪✪✪).

Table 6.2 Summary results of sample trials showing prognostic benefit from statin therapy in patients with coronary disease

Study	Agent	Initial total cholesterol (mmol/l)	Absolute (relative) mortality reduction (%)	Dose (mg)
4 S	Simvastatin	5.5–8.0	4 (30)	10–40
CARE	Pravastatin	<6.2	3 (24)	40

The National Service Framework for Coronary Heart Disease in England recommends that statins and dietary advice be used to lower serum cholesterol concentrations EITHER to less than 5 mmol/l (LDL to below 3 mmol/l) OR by 30%, whichever is the greater.

REFERENCES

107. Carlsson R et al (1995) Serum lipids four weeks after acute myocardial infarction are a valid basis for lipid lowering intervention in patients receiving thrombolysis *Brit Heart J* 74:18–20 (✓)

108. Anonymous (1996) Management of hyperlipidaemia *Drug Ther Bull* 34:57–60 (✓✓✓)

6.6 Nitrates

Despite beneficial symptomatic and pharmacological effects, there is little convincing evidence that nitrate therapy in acute MI carries significant prognostic benefit.

In GISSI-3 there was some evidence of an additive benefit on 6 week mortality when intravenous and then transdermal nitrates were combined with lisinopril. ISIS-4 showed no evidence of a beneficial effect. Meta-analysis of all randomised trials where nitrates were used in the treatment of acute MI have shown a small advantage equivalent to only 4 lives saved/1000 patients treated.

Importantly, there is no evidence of a *detrimental* effect on mortality. Nitrates therefore remain valuable adjunctive therapy for angina, heart failure or severe hypertension post MI.

In other acute coronary syndromes intravenous nitrates remain first-line therapy.

RECOMMENDATIONS

IV nitrates are useful for
1. myocardial ischaemia post-MI (see sections 2.4.4 and 5.1.4.1)
2. unstable angina (see section 5.1.4.1)
3. reduction of high BP prior to planned thrombolysis
4. treatment of left ventricular failure (see section 2.4.1).

The pharmacology of nitrates is succinctly reviewed in reference 111.

REFERENCE

109. Parker JD and Parker JO (1998) Nitrate therapy for stable angina pectoris *NEJM* 338:520–531 (✓✓✓)

6.7 Inotropes

Patients react differently to inotropic drugs and recommended doses represent only a range. There is much to be said for considering clinical end-points such as systolic BP, cardiac output, mean arterial pressure or systemic vascular resistance and adjusting the choice of agent and dose to achieve these end-points.

6.7.1 Dobutamine

Dobutamine is a synthetic molecule derived from isoprenaline with virtually identical haemodynamic effects, namely essentially pure beta-1 agonism. Unlike dopamine it does not cause peripheral vasoconstriction.
Half-life is 2.5 min.

Usual dosage range is 2.5–10 µg/kg/min but the maximum can be increased to 20 or even 30 µg/kg/min in extremis.

It is a positive inotrope, a less strong positive chronotrope and possesses both pulmonary and systemic arterial vasodilator properties. Thus, it reduces both systemic vascular resistance and pulmonary capillary wedge pressure.

Predictably, since it is a catecholamine-like molecule it is pro-arrhythmic but its short plasma half-life limits this problem.

6.7.2 Dopamine

Dopamine has complex pharmacological actions which are partly dose dependent. It is a positive inotrope of similar potency to dobutamine but typically causes only a modest increase in heart rate.
At concentrations below 5 µg/kg/min ('renal' dose) it increases splanchnic blood flow by stimulating dopaminergic receptors and this may promote urine output in an oliguric patient. At higher doses its peripheral vasoconstricting properties become more apparent. Partly for this reason it tends to be used in the UK more to improve renal blood flow at low doses than as a sole inotrope. In the USA dopamine is commonly used as first choice inotrope in doses up to 20 µg/kg/min (ACC/AHA).

Wherever possible intravenous inotropes should be given via a central vein. Short-term peripheral infusion is acceptable as a holding measure while central venous access is being secured.

The pharmacology of dobutamine is reviewed in reference 109.

REFERENCE

110. Sonnenblick EH et al (1979) Dobutamine: a new synthetic cardioactive sympathetic amine *NEJM* 300:17–22 (✓✓✓).

6.7.3 Combination therapy with dobutamine and dopamine

Dobutamine and dopamine are the preferred inotropes in most CCU settings since they have little tendency to increase myocardial oxygen consumption with the possible consequence of increasing infarct size.

A logical and commonly used combination of these agents is in a situation with low systemic BP and oliguria secondary to this. Typically a 'renal' dose of dopamine (e.g. 2–5 µg/kg/min) would be given with a dose of dobutamine (2–10 µg/kg/min although 10–20 µg/kg/min is sometimes required) titrated e.g. to give a systolic BP of >100 mmHg.

6.7.4 Adrenaline (epinephrine)

Adrenaline (epinephrine) is relatively rarely used in CCU practice as an infusion since it causes a significant increase in heart rate and myocardial oxygen consumption, and can provoke malignant arrhythmias. Empirically some patients with hyoptension secondary to poor pump function do respond to adrenaline when dobutamine and/or dopamine has failed, and it may find a use in such patients. As well as the effect on heart rate adrenaline (epinephrine) increases stroke volume, cardiac output and mean arterial pressure. Usual dose range is 1–70 µg/min.

6.7.5 Noradrenaline (norepinephrine)

Noradrenaline (norepinephrine) is rarely useful as a single inotropic agent and finds infrequent use in the CCU.

Pharmacologically it is an alpha-agonist with some beta-1 activity, and acts as a nearly pure vasoconstrictor. Its major role is in severe hypotension where systemic vascular resistance is normal, or in the rare cases where it is low.

European guidelines advise its use in cardiogenic shock with systolic BP <80 mmHg; ACC/AHA guidelines recommend its use where dopamine in doses of up to 20 µg/kg/min has failed to correct a BP <90 mmHg.

Typical doses of noradrenaline (norepinephrine) are 2–20 µg/min. Up to 70 µg/min may be required to achieve pre-set clinical end-points.

Most clinical trials reporting experience with these agents have included very small numbers of patients, often fewer than 20. Overall clinical experience is however vast and these agents remain the first choice inotropes in most CCUs in the UK.

For both adrenaline (epinephrine) and noradrenaline (norepinephrine), if 6 mg of drug is made up in 100 ml 5% dextrose solution then infusion rate in ml/h is approximately equal to delivered dose in µg/min.

6.7.5 Phosphodiesterase inhibitors

Milrinone and enoximone are phosphodiesterase inhibitors and are unusual in combining a positive inotropic effect with vasodilation.

Phosphodiesterase inhibitors may have a particular role where catecholamines cause unacceptable tachycardias or arrhythmias. A 24 h infusion of milrinone has been shown to confer significant haemodynamic improvement at 0.5 µg/kg/min[110].

Milrinone accumulates in patients with renal dysfunction. Usual dose range is 50 µg/kg loading dose and maintenance dose of 0.25–0.75 µg/kg/min.

For enoximone the loading dose is 0.5–1.0 mg/kg with a maintenance dose of 5–10 µg/kg/min.

REFERENCES

111. Klocke RK et al (1991) Effects of a twenty-four-hour milrinone infusion in patients with severe heart failure and cardiogenic shock as a function of the hemodynamic initial condition *Am Heart J* 121:1965–1973 (✓)

6.8 Anti-thrombins and oral anti-coagulants

6.8.1 Heparin

Heparin treament aims to prevent formation of new intravascular thrombus in acute MI, particularly at the site of the ruptured plaque in the infarct-related artery and e.g. in leg veins, during the period of relative immobility. Both unfractionated (UFH) and low molecular weight (LMWH) heparins are now in routine clinical use. Anti-coagulant treatment is a balance between successfully preventing new clot formation or extension, and avoiding bleeds associated with over-treatment.

6.8.1.1 Recommendations for heparin treatment
ACC/AHA Class IIa recommendations (✪✪)
1. IV for 48 h following tPA treatment. Keep APTT 1.5–2.0.
2. IV UFH or SC LMWH for patients with non-ST elevation MI.
3. SC UFH (e.g. 7500 U BD) or LMWH (e.g. enoxaparin 7500 U BD) in all patients not treated with thrombolytics who do not have a contra-indication to heparin.
   Use IV heparin in patients who are at high risk for systemic emboli (large or anterior MI, AF, previous embolus or known LV thrombus).
4. IV UFH in patients treated with thrombolytic agents and who are at high risk for systemic emboli (large or anterior MI, AF, previous embolus or known LV thrombus). It is recommended that heparin be withheld for 4–6 h and then re-started when APTT<2.0 (about 70 s). Keep APTT 1.5 to 2.0. After 48 h, a change to subcutaneous heparin, warfarin, or aspirin alone should be considered.

6.8.1.2 Recommended cautions with heparin treatment
1. Over-anti-coagulation carries significant hazards, particularly of intracranial haemorrhage or other major bleeds. Do not make educated guesses as to dosages – use a locally approved table or nomogram.
2. Heparin-induced thrombocytopaenia (HIT) occurs in up to 3% of patients, and is associated with an increased frequency of **thrombotic** events.

3. Check FBC daily while on IV heparin. If platelet count falls below 100,000, consult with specialist haematologist to exclude or treat HIT and treat patient as being at high risk of thrombotic complications.

4. Concurrent IV nitrate therapy may reduce sensitivity to heparin, requiring dose increases and potential 'rebound' APTT increase when nitrates are stopped.

6.8.2 Warfarin

Warfarin is virtually the only coumadin anti-coagulant used in the UK although acenocoumarol (nicoumalone) and phenindione are also available. Warfarin acts by blocking vitamin K dependent synthesis of clotting factors II, VII, IX and X, and of protein C and protein S. Dosage requirements vary widely between individuals which necessitates individual dosing based on INR, often after one or two initial doses of 10 mg/day.

The use of warfarin in CCU management is to prevent both arterial and venous thrombosis and pulmonary or systemic embolism. Early prophylactic use of heparin and early mobilisation should considerably reduce the risk of these complications and ensure the risks and inconvenience of warfarin therapy are undertaken only when the benefits outweigh these factors. In one study the incidence of serious bleeds was 0.6% per year on warfarin treatment[112].

6.8.2.1 Recommendations for warfarin therapy after MI

1. Left ventricular thrombus (❸❸❸).
2. Paroxysmal or sustained atrial fibrillation (❸❸).
3. Anterior MI with large anterior akinetic segment (❸❸).

In these contexts a target INR of 2.0–3.0 is sufficient.

ACC/AHA guidelines also recommend warfarinisation in post MI patients unable to take daily aspirin, but this is not routine practice in the UK (**Class I recommendation (❸❸❸)**.

There is conflicting evidence about the **routine** use of warfarin post MI. In one randomised study 1214 patients were followed for a mean of 37 months post MI, taking either warfarin or placebo. Deaths, re-infarction and total cerebrovascular accidents were reduced in the group taking warfarin[112]. Another angiographically based study of 300 patients found no superiority of warfarin over aspirin in preventing coronary re-occlusion within 3 months of an MI[113].

REFERENCES

112. Smith P et al (1990) The effect of warfarin on mortality and reinfarction after myocardial infarction. *NEJM* 323:147–152 (✓✓✓)
113. Meijer A et al (1993) Aspirin versus coumadin in the prevention of reocclusion and recurrent ischaemia after successful thrombolysis: a prospective placebo-controlled angiographic study. Results of the APRICOT study *Circulation* 87:1524–1530 (✓✓)

6.9 Amiodarone

Amiodarone has complex anti-arrhythmic actions. It is generally classified a Vaughan–Williams Class III agent, owing to its potassium channel blocki activity with consequent lengthening of the action potential duration a effective refractory period. It also has a beta-blocker-like effect on the sinus a atrio-ventricular nodes (Class II) and weak sodium and calcium chann blocking activity (Class I and Class IV).

Its pharmacokinetics are also complex. Loading requires a total dose of at le 10 g. It is very lipid soluble and adipose tissue acts as a reservoir, giving it a ve long elimination half-life of 30–40 days, but this can exceed 100 days in obe patients. There is little correlation between serum levels and clinical efficacy b a better correlation exists between side-effects and serum levels. Toxic effe are likely at serum levels >2.5 μg/ml.

Amiodarone potentiates the effect of warfarin and increases serum levels digoxin and anti-arrhythmics such as quinidine, procainamide and flecainic More commonly it can cause significant bradycardias in combination with oth rate-slowing agents such as beta-blockers, verapamil, diltiazem and digoxin.

Uses

1. Prophylaxis of ventricular fibrillation
2. Treatment and prophylaxis of ventricular tachycardia
3. Treatment and prophylaxis of pre-excited atrial fibrillation
4. Treatment and prophylaxis of arrhythmias associated with hypertrophic cardiomyopathy
5. Treatment and prophylaxis of supraventricular tachycardias which are otherwise medically refractory
6. Post-CABG control of supraventricular arrhythmias, expecially atrial fibrillation
7. Adjunctive therapy prior to DC cardioversion of AF

For a detailed review of the pharmacology and uses of amiodarone see reference 114.

REFERENCE

114. Mason JW (1987) Amiodarone *NEJM* 316:455–466.

There has been particular interest in the use of amiodarone post MI in the prophylaxis against ventricular arrhythmias or sudden death. Neither CAMIAT nor EMIAT showed an advantage to amiodarone treatment in terms of mortality in this setting, although presumptive arrhythmic deaths were reduced. Importantly there appeared to be no detrimental effect to prophylactic anti-arrhythmic treatment with amiodarone, unlike in CAST where flecainide was shown to be more dangerous than placebo in a post MI setting.

Its toxic effects are many, and potentially life-threatening:

i.   Thyroid function disturbance
Both hyperthyroidism and hypothyroidism can occur (2–4%). The amiodarone molecule contains a significant amount of iodine and blocks peripheral conversion of T4 to T3. Interpretation of thyroid function tests on chronic amiodarone therapy is potentially problematic and usually requires measurement of TSH, free T4 and free T3. High T3 levels with unequivocally suppressed TSH denote a hyperthyroid state.

ii.   Pulmonary fibrosis (6% overall[115]; 5–15% of patients on 400 mg/d chronically)
This is the most feared complication of amiodarone treatment since it is not always reversible on stopping drug treatment and if established is generally fatal. Routine screening should include review of any change in respiratory symptoms or exercise tolerance.

iii.   Corneal microdeposits (98% of patients on long-term treatment)
Over time these can intervere with vision (1–2%). They can be treated with methylcellulose eye-drops or by stopping the drug.

iv.   Photosensitivity (very common)
Usual practice is to advise patients to avoid direct sunlight, and in sunny conditions to wear a hat, keep arms and legs covered and use 'total' sunblock (Specific Protection Factor at least 20) on exposed skin.

v.   QT interval prolongation and pro-arrhythmic effects
QT interval prolongation with amiodarone is usually beneficial, and only occasionally predisposes to ventricular tachycardia. (For review of this and other pro-arrhythmic effects see reference 116.)

vi.   Miscellaneous toxic effects include constipation, tremor, ataxia, peripheral neuropathy and deranged liver function tests.

The toxicity and side-effect profile of amiodarone are reviewed in reference 117.

Thyroid dysfunction secondary to amiodarone treatment is reviewed in reference 118. The review includes a useful algorithm for the interpretation of thyroid function tests in patients taking amiodarone. They recommend long-term cardiological follow-up for these patients.

REFERENCES

115. Dusman RE et al (1990) Clinical features of amiodarone-induced pulmonary toxicity *Circulation* 82:51–59 (✓✓✓)
116. Hohnloser S et al (1994) Amiodarone-associated proarrhythmic effects. A review with special reference to torsade de pointes tachycardia *Ann Intern Med* 121:529–535 (✓✓✓)
117. Wilson JS and Podrid PJ (1991) Side effects from amiodarone *Am Heart J* 121:158–171 (✓✓✓)
118. Newman CM et al (1998) Amiodarone and the thyroid: a practical guide to the management of thyroid dysfunction induced by amiodarone therapy *Heart* 79:121–127 (✓✓✓)

RECOMMENDATIONS

1. Amiodarone is the drug of first choice for the prophylaxis of life-threatening ventricular arrhythmias in survivors of VT, VF or unwitnessed cardiac arrest not secondary to acute MI (✪✪✪).

2. Amiodarone is rarely justified as a treatment for supraventricular arrhythmias. It should be used for chronic treatment of SVTs only where other medical measures have failed, and other drug(s) proved unsuitable (✪✪✪).

   Most SVTs can be controlled with other single drugs or combinations or can be cured or palliated by ablation following electrophysiological assessment. In cases of SVT it is particularly important to assess the relative risks and benefits of amiodarone therapy and discuss these with the patient (✪✪).

3. Amiodarone should not be a substitute for specialist referral for patients who have VF or VT not associated with the first 12 h post MI (✪✪).

4. Short-term (e.g. 6–12 weeks) therapy with amiodarone may be useful for AF occurring post CABG and prior to DC cardioversion or after a failed cardioversion if a further attempt is planned (✪).

5. Patients on amiodarone should be monitored long-term for changes in thyroid, hepatic and respiratory function. This will require a combination of clinical, biochemical and functional assessment (✪✪✪).

Other emergencies in CCU

7.1 Tachycardias

Introduction

Management of tachycardias causes undue anxiety in many junior medical staff. Although detailed descriptions of tachycardias and their management are beyond the scope of this manual, the vast majority of tachycardias can be satisfactorily managed on the basis of a few principles (see below).

This chapter concentrates on the acute management of arrhythmias.

> **PRINCIPLE 1**
> Any tachycardia with haemodynamic compromise should be DC cardioverted without delay
>
> **PRINCIPLE 2**
> The default diagnosis of regular broad-complex tachycardia should be VT
>
> **PRINCIPLE 3**
> The default diagnosis of irregular broad-complex tachycardia should be pre-excited AF
>
> **PRINCIPLE 4**
> Narrow complex tachycardias are all supraventricular in origin. These can safely be treated by slowing AV nodal conduction.
>
> **PRINCIPLE 5**
> ECGs are easy to fax and there is always an expert at the end of a phone.
>
> **PRINCIPLE 6**
> Any survivor of spontaneous VT or resuscitated VF should be referred to an electrophysiologist

In general the objectives of tachycardia management are as follows:

1. Resuscitation of the compromised patient
2. Conversion to sinus rhythm where possible
3. Slowing of the ventricular rate where conversion to sinus rhythm is not possible
4. Removal or correction of the arrhythmic substrate
5. Prevention of recurrence

7.1.1 PRINCIPLE 1
Any tachycardia with haemodynamic compromise should be DC cardioverted without delay

Haemodynamic compromise includes hypotension (usually defined as systolic BP < 90 mmHg), angina or impaired consciousness.

If the patient is unconscious with VT the decision to cardiovert is easy since the situation effectively becomes a cardiac arrest. However, this principle also applies to fast AF and atrial flutter where the patient is compromised. Other narrow-complex tachycardias may be treated with IV adenosine, but if this fails DC cardioversion should be the next option.

A conscious, but uncomfortable, and hypotensive patient will represent an unattractive proposition to the on-call anaesthetist. None the less, tachycardia with haemodynamic compromise is a medical emergency requiring prompt treatment under anaesthetic. It is helpful if CCU medical staff and anaesthetists agree guidelines to manage such situations before they arise.

DC cardioversion of rhythms other than VF should be performed with shocks **synchronised** to the ECG. Energies as low as 50 J may be enough to cardiovert some rhythms. With AF the first shock should be given at 200 J and increased to 360 J if unsuccessful. At least 2 shocks should be given at maximum energy before deciding that cardioversion has been unsuccessful.

7.1.2 PRINCIPLE 2
The default diagnosis of regular broad-complex tachycardia
should be VT

Tachycardias can be usefully classified as broad or narrow complex, depending on whether the QRS complex exceeds 0.12 s or not (3 small squares on standard ECG).

Broad-complex tachycardias (BCT) are usually VT. Narrow-complex tachycardias are never VT. However, if an SVT is conducted to the ventricles in the presence of a BBB the complexes will appear broad, as they do in sinus rhythm with bundle branch block. Hence, a few SVTs can present as BCT. This group is usually referred to as SVT with aberrant conduction, the 'aberration' being the bundle-branch block. Unfortunately this relatively rare group of tachycardias is frequently over-diagnosed. This has grave practical consequences if verapamil is given to abort a presumed SVT since this can cause asystole or catastrophic hypotension if the rhythm is VT.

Inaccurate diagnosis will in any case compromise the possibility of successful treatment, particularly in an emergency.

Clinical and ECG criteria will generally allow VT to be distinguished from other BCTs. In VT, with rare exceptions, there is complete AV dissociation so that every so often the right atrium will contract against a closed tricuspid valve. This causes intermittent cannon 'a' waves in the JVP and a first heart sound varying in intensity from beat to beat. These features can be reliably used to determine the presence of VT (see Table 7.2)

> If the patient has coronary artery disease, a broad-complex tachycardia is likely to be VT at least 95% of the time

ECG distinction of SVT from VT in broad complex tachycardia is important, but not always obvious. The proposal that unless SVT could be diagnosed by fulfilling simple criteria, then VT should be accepted as the default diagnosis was first validated by Griffith and colleagues[119]. The criterion for SVT was the finding of **typical** bundle branch block patterns (see Table 7.1)

Table 7.1 Criteria for typical left and right bundle branch block

Left bundle	rS or QS in leads V1 and V2 delay to S wave nadir <70 ms R wave and no Q wave in lead V6
Right bundle	rSR' wave in lead V1 RS wave in lead V6 with R wave height greater than S wave depth

Using only these criteria the sensitivity for detecting VT was 90% and this rose to 96% when independent P waves (diagnostic of VT) were sought in cases thought to be SVT.

Table 7.2 Clinical utility of JVP and first heart sound in diagnosing VT[120]

	JVP	First heart sound
Specificity	96%	58%
Sensitivity	75%	100%
Positive predictive value	82%	100%

REFERENCES

119. Griffith MJ et al (1994) Ventricular tachycardia as default diagnosis in broad complex tachycardia *Lancet* 343:386–388 (✓)
120. Garratt CJ et al (1994) Value of physical signs in the diagnosis of ventricular tachycardia *Circulation* 90:3103–3107 (✓)

Conclusive proof of VT on the ECG can be found if AV dissociation can be demonstrated by finding

1. Evidence of independent P wave activity which will be at a slower rate than the QRS complexes
2. 'Capture' beats which are intermittent narrow-complex beats preceded by a P wave
3. 'Fusion' beats where a P wave can be seen superimposed on a wide QRS complex

One or other of these features is seen in only a minority of cases, probably 20–30%.

Further helpful, but not conclusive, criteria include

> Taller initial R wave (RSr') in V1
> Frontal QRS axis in 'no-man's land' i.e. +180° to +270°
> QR or RS wave in V1
> rS or QS wave in V6
> Concordance of QRS polarity in all chest leads

> The combination of clinical examination and ECG analysis should therefore allow a definitive diagnosis in at least 95% of cases of VT

RECOMMENDATIONS

1. Assume BCT is VT unless there is **overwhelming** evidence to the contrary (❸❸❸).
2. If the patient is unstable, DC cardiovert (❸❸❸) (**Principle 1**).
3. If the patient is stable and there is a question of the rhythm being SVT give adenosine 6–12 mg IV. This will have no effect on VT but will slow or abort an SVT. If no effect proceed to treatment as for VT (❸❸❸).
4. VT can be treated with (❸❸❸)

   i.   Sotalol 1.5 mg/kg IV (70 kg patient ~100 mg)

   ii. Lignocaine 1 mg/kg IV max 100 mg as IV bolus

   iii. Procainamide 100 mg IV over 1–5 min, repeated up to maximum of 1–1.5 g

   iv. Amiodarone 150–300 mg IV over 10–60 min, followed by 900 mg over 24 h

   v.   Overdrive pacing (see opposite).

Many of these criteria are different facets of the criteria used to diagnose 'typical' bundle branch block in Table 7.1.

Concordance means 'pointing the same way'. If all complexes point up this suggests a tachycardia originating in the LV, if all point down this indicates RV tachycardia.

Sotalol has been shown in a small randomised trial to be superior to lignocaine as a first line agent to abort spontaneous sustained VT[121].

There little or no prospective randomised data to support the use of procainamide or amiodarone over other agents in this setting.

Overdrive pacing

The aim is to interrupt the tachycardia by making the ventricle refractory as the next beat of tachycardia is due. A right ventricular pacing wire is used. Pace at a rate ~50/min above the tachycardia rate. Ensure pacing is 'capturing' the ventricle. Stop pacing after 5–10 s. If no response increase the pacing rate by 10/min, e.g. from 210 to 220/min and repeat. In general it is worth several attempts pacing within the range 180–240/min. Do not pace at rates higher than 250/min – it is safer to proceed to DC cardioversion.

REFERENCES

121. Ho DS et al (1994) Double-blind trial of lignocaine versus sotalol for acute termination of spontaneous sustained ventricular tachycardia *Lancet* 344:18–23 (✓)

Treatment of recurrent VT

Many tachycardias have a primary underlying cause or precipitant and some of these may be reversible, including

> myocardial ischaemia
> electrolyte abnormalities (includes calcium and magnesium)
> drug-induced long QT syndrome
> pro-arrhythmic effect of anti-arrhythmic treatment
> trauma
> endocrine disorders e.g. thyrotoxicosis

Non-reversible causes include

> left ventricular aneurysm
> right ventricular dysplasia
> congenital long QT syndromes
> malignant infiltration of myocardium or pericardium
> congenital structural heart disease with or without surgical correction

RECOMMENDATIONS

1. Reverse or treat any potential precipitating cause (✪✪✪).
2. Beta-blockers, particularly sotalol, are useful if ischaemia is likely to be contributing to any VT (✪✪✪).
3. VT which has responded to lignocaine is likely to respond to oral mexiletine (✪).
4. Amiodarone is probably the best choice of agent for VT associated with haemodynamic instability or requiring out-of-hospital resuscitation. Amiodarone is useful in patients with poor LV function since it has little significant negative inotropy (✪✪✪).

Treatment of recurrent VT in patients with poor ventricular function remains a challenge and is best managed by a specialist. Anti-arrhythmic combinations which may prove useful include

> amiodarone plus beta-blockers
> amiodarone plus mexiletine
> sotalol plus mexiletine

The pharmacokinetics of amiodarone demand a large loading dose of approximately 10 g. This is conveniently given as 400 mg TDS for 8 days although any initial IV dose can be counted in the total. Maintenance dose is 200 mg/day PO. There is no advantage to giving higher doses chronically and toxic effects are more likely (see section 6.6)

7.1.3 PRINCIPLE 3
The default diagnosis of irregular broad-complex tachycardia should be pre-excited AF

An irregular BCT is usually AF conducted with BBB. However, it is much more dangerous to ignore the possibility of 'pre-excited' AF where the earliest activation of the ventricles is via one or more accessory pathways (as in Wolff–Parkinson–White syndrome) since this can lead to VF. The reason for this is that accessory pathways are often capable of rapid 'non-decremental' conduction and unlike the AV node can still conduct 1:1 at very high supraventricular rates. Thus AF, with effective atrial rates of 400/min or more, can be conducted directly to the ventricles, causing VF. Treatment of pre-excited AF with AV nodal blocking agents such as digoxin or verapamil is likely to exacerbate matters since this encourages all conduction to go down the accessory pathway(s). Despite their AV nodal blocking action beta-blockers such as sotalol appear to be safe, since they also block conduction in the accessory pathway.

In a manner analogous to diagnosing regular broad-complex tachycardia it should be assumed that an irregular BCT is pre-excited AF, unless a **typical** bundle-branch block pattern can be demonstrated (see Table 7.1).

RECOMMENDATIONS

1. Acute treatment of pre-excited AF
   DC cardioversion if unstable (**Principle 1**)
   IV flecainide 2 mg/kg slow injection with ECG and BP monitoring
   Amiodarone 150–300 mg IV over 60 min, then 900 mg over 24 h, followed by oral loading.
2. Preventing recurrence of pre-excited AF
   Flecainide 50–150 mg/day PO in divided doses
   Amiodarone 200 mg/day PO after initial loading.

> All patients with ventricular pre-excitation should be referred to an electrophysiologist for consideration for invasive study and/or ablation of the accessory pathway(s)

A 12 lead ECG taken in sinus rhythm will usually reveal a short PR interval and delta waves in some of the QRS complexes confirming the diagnosis of pre-excitation.

However if an accessory pathway conducts antegradely (i.e. from atrium to ventricle) only intermittently these may be absent.

When giving IV anti-arrhythmic agents

1. Monitor the patient's ECG
2. Monitor the patient's BP
3. Do not be tempted to give 'slow boluses' faster than recommended
4. Be prepared to resuscitate a patient who becomes hypotensive or who develops significant bradycardia or tachycardia

> **7.1.4 PRINCIPLE 4**
> Narrow complex tachycardias are all supraventricular in origin. These can safely be treated by slowing AV nodal conduction

Carotid sinus massage or other vagotonic manoeuvres are worth trying prior to drugs. The success of such manoeuvres is augmented if the patient performs a concurrent Valsalva manoeuvre.

Adenosine is the first choice drug treatment. It acts as an AV nodal blocker with the advantage of a very short half-life (1–5 s). AV nodal blockade is likely to abort a tachycardia involving the AV node in a circuit. It will have little effect on tachycardias resulting from discharge of an automatic focus, although some true atrial tachycardias may be terminated by adenosine. Adenosine will also be ineffective at aborting AF or atrial flutter, although it may slow the ventricular response transiently.

Since adenosine is directly metabolised within seconds there are virtually no disadvantages to its use. The manufacturers recommended that it be avoided in asthmatic patients, though there are few reports of this being a problem in practice. Its half-life is prolonged in patients taking dipyridamole.

Acute treatment of NCTs is directed at restoring sinus rhythm, but if this is not possible then controlling the ventricular response is the next goal.

The advantage of longer-acting AV nodal blockers is that if the tachycardia cannot be aborted then the ventricular response rate can generally be controlled.

RECOMMENDATIONS

1. Adenosine should be tried as first-choice agent in all regular NCTs at doses from 6 to 18 mg as a fast IV bolus (✪✪✪).
2. If adenosine is ineffective ventricular rate slowing should be achieved using AV nodal blocking agents (✪✪ – see below).
3. If there is a firm diagnosis of AF or atrial flutter adenosine should not be used as it will not be effective (✪✪✪).

There is a rare exception to Principle 4. So-called fascicular tachycardia can show complexes <0.12 s with a morphology similar to RBBB. However, the complexes generally show a small initial q wave rather than a large R wave. There is associated left axis deviation. This tachycardia is generally sensitive to treatment with verapamil.

AV nodal blocking agents include

1. Beta-blockers
2. Digoxin
3. Verapamil
4. Diltiazem

Esmolol has been advocated as a very short-acting beta-blocker for use as an anti-arrhythmic. In practice the administration regimen is rather complex and it is usually at least as convenient to give slow IV boluses of 40 mg of sotalol up to a maximum of 120–160 mg.

Digoxin is a poor anti-arrhythmic but a reasonable AV nodal blocker. It is positively inotropic. An IV or PO loading dose of 1 mg, given as 2×500 mcg doses 4–6 h apart is usually sufficient, with a chronic dose of 0.25 mg OD in patients of average build and normal renal function.

Verapamil can be given as 5 mg IV aliquots up to a total of 15 mg if beta-blockers cannot be used.

Verapamil should NOT be given to anyone who has recently received beta-blockers, **or if there is any chance that a rhythm is VT**.

Diltiazem is rarely used as an anti-arrhythmic, but depending on the clinical context may offer some useful AV nodal slowing as an adjunct to its anti-ischaemic effects.

When giving IV anti-arrhythmic agents

1. Monitor the patient's ECG
2. Monitor the patient's BP
3. Do not be tempted to give 'slow boluses' faster than recommended
4. Be prepared to resuscitate a patient who becomes hypotensive or who develops significant bradycardia or tachycardia

In a review of AF treatment diltiazem was found to have no benefit in AF other than rate slowing[122].

REFERENCE

122. Pritchett ELC (1992) Management of atrial fibrillation *NEJM* 326:1264–1271 (✓✓✓)

> ### 7.1.5 PRINCIPLE 5
> ECGs are easy to fax and there is always an expert at the end of a phone

ECGs lend themselves very well to fax or electronic transmission and it should always be possible to contact the responsible local consultant, or the relevant tertiary cardiac centre, and obtain advice about diagnosis and management.

Ideally a 12-lead ECG in tachycardia and in sinus rhythm (or other usual rhythm) should be made available. Individual CCUs are likely to have established links with a tertiary centre for advice and for transfers of emergencies.

> ### 7.1.6 PRINCIPLE 6
> Any survivor of an out-of-hospital cardiac arrest or of spontaneous sustained VT should be referred to an electrophysiologist

These patients may require a combination of therapies including coronary revascularisation, anti-arrhythmics and an implantable defibrillator.

7.2 Bradycardias

The management of bradycardias which cause symptoms sufficient to warrant hospital admission is usually straightforward. If a reversible cause cannot be identified the patient is likely to need permanent pacing. Essentially three questions need to be addressed

1. Is there a reversible cause of the bradycardia?

2. Is temporary pacing required, until the cause can be reversed, or until permanent pacing can be arranged?

3. Is permanent pacing required?

Reversible causes

These are relatively few and include

Electrolyte disturbances, particularly extreme values of serum potassium

Hypothyrodism

Unsuspected or recent myocardial infarction

Overdose of rate-slowing drugs (iatrogenic, deliberate or accidental)

Failure of a permanent pacing system

Temporary pacing

Temporary pacing should be **avoided** unless the patient is hypotensive (e.g. BP <90 mmHg with symptoms), symptomatic or shows other signs of cardiac dysfunction or vital organ hypoperfusion attributable to the bradycardia.

Temporary transvenous pacing has a high complication rate when performed by non-specialists or the relatively inexperienced[123] and is associated with a higher level of infection of subsequently implanted permanent pacing systems.

Permanent pacing

Patients with symptomatic bradycardias with non-reversible causes should be referred for permanent pacemaker implant. Rhythms requiring referral in any case include

Complete heart block

2nd degree heart block of any type

Sinus arrest

Bradycardia–tachycardia syndrome

Ventricular standstill

REFERENCE

123. Connaughton M et al (1998) The learning curve for temporary pacing: evidence from district general and teaching hospitals *Heart* 79 Supp 1 P51 (✓)

RECOMMENDATIONS

1. Serum electrolytes, magnesium and calcium should be measured in any patient presenting with bradycardia. Thyroid function should be checked clinically and biochemically (✪✪✪).

2. A 12 lead ECG and long (30–60 s) rhythm strip should be taken (✪✪✪).

3. Recent myocardial infarction should be excluded by history and ECG examination, and if necessary by measure of serum markers (✪✪✪).

4. A thorough drug history should be taken. If the patient is too unwell, relatives or a carer may be able to help.
   Do not forget the possibility of deliberate drug overdose (✪✪✪).

5. Perform a well-penetrated chest X-ray if the patient already has a permanent pacing system. This can reveal such problems as lead fracture and lead tip displacement. Arrange for early interrogation of the pacing system (✪✪✪).

6. Insert an RV pacing lead if the patient requires pacing prior to transfer for implant of a permanent system or until appropriate treatment can be completed to reverse the bradycardia (✪✪✪).

7.3 Pacemakers

7.3.1 Introduction

Although a pacemaker is a complex system the hardware consists only of two components, the generator and lead(s). Failure can occur only in one or other of these, at the interface between them, or at the interface between the pacing system and myocardium.

Nearly all rhythm problems secondary to pacing system malfunction can be understood in terms of

1. failure to pace, either at all, or appropriately
2. failure to sense, either at all, or appropriately.

With minimal knowledge of pacing systems, a 12 lead ECG, a CXR and a magnet most pacemaker problems can be analysed.

When seeking specialist advice aim to answer the following questions:

1. Ideally, what is the manufacturer and model of the pacing system?
2. What is the pacing mode of the system e.g. VVIR, DDD?
3. Is there evidence of a strictly mechanical problem?
4. Is there evidence of sepsis related to the pacing system?
5. Is there 'failure to pace'?
6. Is there 'failure to sense'?

7.3.2 Pacing modes

The standard codes for describing pacing mode are summarised in Table 7.3 opposite.

Thus, a rate-responsive atrial single-chamber system would be denoted AAIR, and a non-rate responsive ventricular system VVI.

Table 7.3 Four-letter codes for describing pacing system mode

First letter Chamber paced	Second letter Chamber sensed	Third letter Response to a sensed beat	Fourth letter Rate-responsiveness
V ventricle	V ventricle	I inhibited	R yes
A atrium	A atrium	T triggered	O no
D A and V	D A and V	D dual	
	O none	O nothing	

7.3.4 Manufacturer, model and pacing mode

Patients usually carry a card with details of the type of pacemaker and pacing mode programmed at the time of implant. Most generators carry a manufacturer's logo and code which allow identification from CXR, although this is rarely required in practice.

With a single atrial lead visible on CXR the pacing mode is almost certainly AAI(R).

With a single ventricular lead, the mode is almost certainly VVI(R), although dual-chamber sensing from a single lead is now possible. This is termed VDI.

If two leads are attached to the generator the system is dual-chamber, usually DDD(R).

7.3.5 Sepsis

The two major septic problems associated with pacing systems are infection associated with generator erosion through the chest wall, or right-sided endocarditis. The former is obvious clinically, the latter is fortunately rare. If there is clinical suspicion of sepsis, right-sided endocarditis should be sought by blood culture, echocardiography and serum inflammatory markers. Any problems thought secondary to sepsis involving a pacing system should be discussed with the local cardiac centre.

7.3.6 Mechanical problems

Well-penetrated PA and lateral chest films will provide good information about the generator-lead interface, the lead, and the lead–myocardium interface. Search specifically for
1. Failure of the lead terminal to be fully engaged with the generator head
2. Lead fracture
3. Discontinuity in lead insulation
4. Unusual position of lead tip, suggesting displacement

Unusual, but appropriate lead tip positions usually require active fixation leads which generally have a small 'corkscrew' at the tip. If this is not visible with an unusual lead tip position assume displacement and look for 'failure to pace'.

7.3.7 Diagnosing 'failure to pace'

1. Place a magnet over the pacemaker generator. This switches it temporarily to 'magnet mode'. The system should then pace at a predetermined rate, irrespective of the heart's underlying activity, e.g. in VOO mode for a ventricular system. The exact 'magnet rate' varies between manufacturers. In a dual chamber system the pacemaker is generally switched to DOO in magnet mode. If the chamber (atrium or ventricle) is not 'captured' by this activity then 'failure to pace' can be diagnosed.
2. A 12 lead ECG and 30–60 s rhythm strip should be examined carefully for pacing spikes. These are very short in duration typically 0.5 ms, and bipolar spikes may have an amplitude of only 1–2 mm in many leads. However, once pacing spikes are located it should be possible to deduce whether capture is achieved when a chamber is paced at any time when it should not be refractory.

7.3.8 Diagnosing 'failure to sense'

This is more difficult, but can be inferred if a pacing spike is seen when it is clearly inappropriate e.g. in the ST-T segment of the ECG, or very shortly after a native QRS.

7.3.9 Pacemaker mediated tachycardia ('Endless loop tachycardia')

This is rare, and all modern devices are designed to minimise its occurrence. In essence, in a dual-chamber pacing system the ventricular lead acts as the antegrade or forward limb of a tachycardia circuit, the retrograde limb comprising conducting tissue e.g. the AV node or an accessory pathway. The tachycardia is easily interrupted by placing a magnet over the generator.

Table 7.4 Common causes of sensing and pacing failure

	Failure to sense	Failure to pace
Generator	Battery end-of-life Inappropriate settings e.g. sensitivity too low Software problem	Battery end-of-life Inappropriate settings e.g. programmed output too low Software problem
Generator-lead connection	Disconnection	Disconnection
Lead	Lead displacement Lead fracture Insulation failure	Lead displacement Lead fracture
Lead-myocardium interface	Myocardial infarction Drug effect Oedema e.g. in myocarditis	Myocardial infarction Drug effect e.g. flecainide

7.4 Automatic implantable cardioverter-defibrillators (AICDs)

> All AICD manufacturers have emergency contact numbers for advice

These devices are now an integral part of the management of life-threatening arrhythmias. As such, district hospital CCUs will all encounter patients with an implant, or problems pertaining to one.

AICD programming and therapy is a subject in itself but management of immediate problems is relatively simple. AICDs are rescue devices designed to prevent sudden cardiac death (SCD). All modern devices are capable of anti-tachycardia (overdrive) pacing, defibrillation and anti-bradycardia pacing. Nearly always the initial programmed therapy will involve anti-tachycardia pacing if VT is detected followed by a cardioverting shock if this fails. A shock will be programmed if the VT is very rapid, or if VF is detected. Successful cardioversion or defibrillation is often followed by asystole or bradycardias, so a requirement for pacing by the AICD following a shock is common. AICDs will also act as an anti-bradycardia pacemaker if a bradycardia develops for any other reason.

In practice, the vast majority of presentations will occur following a shock. The diagnostic problem is straightforward and involves determining whether the shock was appropriate or not. A shock is appropriate therapy if the patient experiences VT not terminated by anti-tachycardia pacing, or develops VF. It is inappropriate if delivered during rhythms other than VT or VF.

If **appropriate**, further management is directed at improving prophylaxis of further arrhythmias. Such therapy may already have been optimised. In such cases it should be accepted that the AICD has performed its role correctly and no further intervention is required.

If **inappropriate** shocks are delivered then the device requires reprogramming or replacement. If multiple or repeated inappropriate shocks are being delivered AICDs can generally be switched off by placing a magnet over the generator box.

Patients who have had their AICD turned off should be regarded as being at continuing risk of SCD. They should be monitored, and be within reach of an external defibrillator, including during transfer to a specialist unit.

RECOMMENDATIONS

1. Any patient who has received a shock from an AICD should initially be monitored on CCU (✪✪✪).
2. Contact the cardiac centre responsible for AICD follow-up and arrange for early device interrogation/re-programming (✪✪✪).
3. Screen for myocardial infarction with serial ECGs (if interpretable) and serum markers (✪✪✪).
4. Rule out or treat any electrolyte imbalance (✪✪✪).
5. Check for drug compliance and intercurrent illness (✪✪✪).
6. If multiple or repeated inappropriate shocks are being delivered switch the AICD off by placing a magnet over the generator box (✪✪✪).